Metal Surfaces

Metal Surfaces

Editors

Roberto Montanari
Saulius Kaciulis

MDPI • Basel • Beijing • Wuhan • Barcelona • Belgrade • Manchester • Tokyo • Cluj • Tianjin

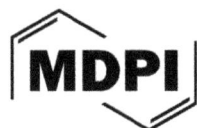

Editors
Roberto Montanari
Universy of Rome "Tor Vergata"
Italy

Saulius Kaciulis
Istituto per lo Studio dei Materiali Nanostrutturati
Italy

Editorial Office
MDPI
St. Alban-Anlage 66
4052 Basel, Switzerland

This is a reprint of articles from the Special Issue published online in the open access journal *Coatings* (ISSN 2079-6412) (available at: https://www.mdpi.com/journal/coatings/special_issues/matal_Surf).

For citation purposes, cite each article independently as indicated on the article page online and as indicated below:

LastName, A.A.; LastName, B.B.; LastName, C.C. Article Title. *Journal Name* **Year**, *Volume Number*, Page Range.

ISBN 978-3-0365-1012-5 (Hbk)
ISBN 978-3-0365-1013-2 (PDF)

© 2021 by the authors. Articles in this book are Open Access and distributed under the Creative Commons Attribution (CC BY) license, which allows users to download, copy and build upon published articles, as long as the author and publisher are properly credited, which ensures maximum dissemination and a wider impact of our publications.

The book as a whole is distributed by MDPI under the terms and conditions of the Creative Commons license CC BY-NC-ND.

Contents

About the Editors vii

Saulius Kaciulis and Roberto Montanari
Metal Surfaces
Reprinted from: *Coatings* 2021, *11*, 255, doi:10.3390/coatings11020255 1

Ishwer Shivakoti, Golam Kibria, Robert Cep, Bal Bahadur Pradhan and Ashis Sharma
Laser Surface Texturing for Biomedical Applications: A Review
Reprinted from: *Coatings* 2021, *11*, 124, doi:10.3390/coatings11020124 5

Eleonora Bolli, Saulius Kaciulis and Alessio Mezzi
ESCA as a Tool for Exploration of Metals' Surface
Reprinted from: *Coatings* 2020, *10*, 1182, doi:10.3390/coatings10121182 21

Eleonora Bolli, Alessandra Fava, Paolo Ferro, Saulius Kaciulis, Alessio Mezzi, Roberto Montanari and Alessandra Varone
Cr Segregation and Impact Fracture in a Martensitic Stainless Steel
Reprinted from: *Coatings* 2020, *10*, 843, doi:10.3390/coatings10090843 49

Cheng Zhang, Pu Li, Hui Dong, Dongliang Jin, Jinfeng Huang, Feng Mao and Chong Chen
Repetitive Impact Wear Behaviors of the Tempered 25Cr3Mo2NiWV Fe-Based Steel
Reprinted from: *Coatings* 2020, *10*, 107, doi:10.3390/coatings10020107 67

Claudio Mele, Francesca Lionetto and Benedetto Bozzini
An Erosion-Corrosion Investigation of Coated Steel for Applications in the Oil and Gas Field, Based on Bipolar Electrochemistry
Reprinted from: *Coatings* 2020, *10*, 92, doi:10.3390/coatings10020092 79

Roberto Montanari, Ekaterina Pakhomova, Riccardo Rossi, Maria Richetta and Alessandra Varone
Surface Morphological Features of Molybdenum Irradiated by a Single Laser Pulse
Reprinted from: *Coatings* 2020, *10*, 67, doi:10.3390/coatings10010067 91

Qiqi Yu, Daosheng Wen, Shouren Wang, Beibei Kong, Shuxu Wu and Teng Xiao
Effect of 0.8 at.% H on the Mechanical Properties and Microstructure Evolution of a Ti–45Al–9Nb Alloy Under Uniaxial Tension at High Temperature
Reprinted from: *Coatings* 2020, *10*, 52, doi:10.3390/coatings10010052 103

Asiful H. Seikh, Muneer Baig, Jitendra Kumar Singh, Jabair A. Mohammed, Monis Luqman, Hany S. Abdo, Amir Rahman Khan and Nabeel H. Alharthi
Microstructural and Corrosion Characteristics of Al-Fe Alloys Produced by High-Frequency Induction-Sintering Process
Reprinted from: *Coatings* 2019, *9*, 686, doi:10.3390/coatings9100686 119

About the Editors

Roberto Montanari is Full Professor of Metallurgy. He was the head of the PhD programme of Industrial Engineering at the University of Rome "Tor Vergata", 2012–2019, and is currently the President of COMET (Council of Italian Academics of Metallurgy), 2014–2021. He has authored about 330 scientific publications covering different topics such as the deformation of metals under shock loads; materials for application in nuclear reactors; the development of innovative indentation tests; and the study of metallic artefacts of archaeological, historical, and artistic interest. His present research fields are: (i) materials used for aerospace applications, (ii) the structure of liquid metals and precursor effects of melting and solidification, (iii) indentation tests, and (iv) surface engineering. The common thread running through his scientific activity is the study of the relations between the microstructure of metals and their mechanical properties. In 2016, he received the THERMEC Distinguished Award.

Saulius Kaciulis graduated in Physics at the University of Vilnius (Lithuania) in 1977 and received his PhD degree from the same university in 1983. At present, he is Director of Research at the Institute for the Study of Nanostructured Materials (ISMN), and is a member of the National Research Council (CNR) of Italy. He is a member of the PhD Commission for Industrial Engineering at the University of Rome "Tor Vergata". He is a member of the international advisory board of ECASIA (European Conference on Applications of Surface and Interface Analysis), as well as a member of the committee for physical metallurgy and materials science of the Italian Association of Metallurgy (AIM). He is a co-author of over 230 scientific publications with a citation index h = 33 (Scopus, 2021). His current research interests fall in the field of the surface analysis and depth profiling of innovative solid-state materials, including thin films and heterostructures, anti-wear and corrosion-resistant coatings, biocompatible materials, and nanostructured and bidimensional materials.

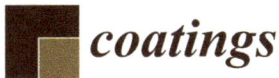

Editorial

Metal Surfaces

Saulius Kaciulis [1,*] and Roberto Montanari [2]

1. Institute for the Study of Nanostructured Materials, ISMN-CNR, P.O. Box 10, 00015 Monterotondo Stazione, 00133 Rome, Italy
2. Department of Industrial Engineering, University of Rome "Tor Vergata", Via del Politecnico 1, 00133 Rome, Italy; roberto.montanari@uniroma2.it
* Correspondence: saulius.kaciulis@cnr.it

1. Introduction and Scope

Surface phenomena such as corrosion, wear, heterogeneous catalysis, segregation, etc., have great relevance in a lot of industrial processes and products. In recent years, the surface structure and chemistry of and the surface phenomena occurring in metals, in particular segregation, oxidation, surface defects and implants, and their reactions with the human body have attracted increasing attention from many investigators. Therefore, quite a bit of scientific work has been devoted to the matter and the results contributed to deepen basic knowledge, improve industrial products and develop new industrial applications. Great attention has been paid to new coatings and processes able to functionalize the metal surface (surface engineering) so that it can play an active role towards the surrounding environment.

In addition to the more conventional characterization techniques, such as electron microscopies, X-ray diffraction (XRD), etc., advanced surface-sensitive techniques such as X-ray photoelectron spectroscopy (XPS), Auger electron spectroscopy (AES) and electron energy loss spectroscopy (EELS) have also been widely applied for studying various metals and their alloys.

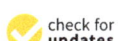

This editorial collects both review and research papers focused on metals' surface and presents investigations in different areas of physics, chemistry, materials science and engineering. The scope is to highlight the state of the art and the latest achievements in this research field. The main topics include:

- Physical and chemical phenomena on the surface;
- Surface morphology and structure;
- Surface modifications and treatments;
- Thin coatings.

Citation: Kaciulis, S.; Montanari, R. Metal Surfaces. *Coatings* **2021**, *11*, 255. https://doi.org/10.3390/coatings11020255

Received: 18 February 2021
Accepted: 19 February 2021
Published: 22 February 2021

Publisher's Note: MDPI stays neutral with regard to jurisdictional claims in published maps and institutional affiliations.

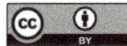

Copyright: © 2021 by the authors. Licensee MDPI, Basel, Switzerland. This article is an open access article distributed under the terms and conditions of the Creative Commons Attribution (CC BY) license (https://creativecommons.org/licenses/by/4.0/).

2. Contributions

The present editorial consists of two reviews [1,2] and six research papers [3–8] dealing with different metals and their properties, which were investigated by various techniques.

The review paper by Shivakoti et al. [1] describes the technique of laser surface texturing (LST) for biomedical applications. Recent developments in LST led to drastic improvements of efficient biomaterials and demonstrated the strong potential of the technique for surface modifications and successful applications of modified materials in the biomedical field. Among the methods for generating textures or patterns on a metal surface, the paper focuses the attention on texturing using laser ablation and texturing using laser interference. Various types of lasers, such as carbon dioxide, excimer, fiber laser, etc., have been used to produce texture and explore the efficacy of the process and its impact on proliferation, osteo-integration and cell adhesion. Specific applications to Ti and its alloys, zirconia, magnesium alloys, Co–Cr–Mo alloys, Cu, austenitic stainless steels and polymers are presented and critically discussed.

The second review by Bolli et al. [2] is devoted to the applications of surface-sensitive spectroscopies (XPS and AES) described by the term Electron Spectroscopy for Chemical Analysis (ESCA). The main principles of ESCA are briefly introduced and its applications for the characterization of various metals and their coatings are illustrated by numerous experimental cases, including, also, scanning photoelectron microscopy (SPEM) by using synchrotron radiation. The reported examples comprise the study of defects on the surface of precious metals, the chemical distribution in Ni-based superalloys after various heat treatments, nitride coatings on stainless steel, composites of Ti6Al4V alloy reinforced by SiC fibers and graphene interface with electrodeposited metal films.

One of the research papers presents an investigation of Cr segregation in a martensitic stainless steel and its effect on fracture [3]. The examined steel is considered to be of interest for structural applications in future nuclear fusion reactors. The fracture surfaces of samples treated in two different conditions (as-quenched and quenched plus annealed) and broken in Charpy tests were examined by XPS. The dependence of Fe/Cr ratio on the test temperature revealed the segregation of Cr in microscopic zones, representing weaker spots in the steel matrix and a preferential path for moving cracks. This study evidenced how Cr segregation is playing a role not only in the intergranular mode of fracture but also in the quasi-cleavage and ductile ones. The results have been related to the formation of C–Cr associates on an atomic scale and their evolution. Another interesting finding presented in this work was obtained by small-area XPS measurements. They revealed that the Fe/Cr ratio is not constant across the surface, being lower in the inner part of the probe. Finite Element Method (FEM) simulations showed that this phenomenon is due to a slower cooling rate in the inner part of Charpy probes, with a consequently longer random walk of diffusing atoms.

The wear behavior of tempered 25Cr3Mo2NiWV steel has been described in the paper of Zhang et al. [4]. Impact wear tests were performed with a dynamic abrasive wear tester on the material previously submitted to various heat treatments for generating different mechanical properties. Both the hardness and toughness affect the wear properties of this steel; namely, the best combination of hardness and toughness corresponds to the lowest wear weight loss. Moreover, the results show that by increasing the wear time, the dominant wear mechanism changes from slight plastic deformation to micro-cutting and adhesive wear, and micro fatigue peeling finally occurs. Fatigue cracks initiate from the surface or the sub-surface and then propagate and converge to form fatigue delamination. SEM observations of cracks in the cross-section demonstrate that brittle fatigue cracks are mainly present in the steels with higher hardness, whereas the ductile fatigue ones occur in the steels with high toughness.

Erosion–corrosion problems of carbon steels, materials of interest for application in the oil and gas field, have been investigated through a bipolar electrochemistry technique by Mele et al. [5]. Steel samples were coated with high phosphorus electroless Ni (ENP) and with a thermo-sprayed coating, consisting of a Ni-based hard alloy with chromium boride dispersion, obtained with the high velocity oxy fuel (HVOF) technique. For comparison, the same experiments were carried out on uncoated steel. The paper demonstrates the suitability of this simple, contactless technique for effective discrimination of the erosion–corrosion behavior of different coatings in working conditions. Through polarization curves, visual inspection and SEM morphological analysis, the effects due to erosion–corrosion by solid particles and by fluid and those due to simple erosion were evaluated.

The modifications of surface morphology in Mo irradiated by a single laser pulse delivered by a Nd:YAG/Glass laser are reported in [6]. Mo is considered as a plasma-facing material alternative to W in the divertor armors of the International Thermonuclear Experimental Reactor (ITER). Transient high energy loads occurring in a tokamak were simulated by a high-intensity single laser pulse and the induced changes were examined by SEM observations. An erosion crater forms in the central area of the irradiated zone due to metal vaporization and the ejection of molten metal. The thermal gradient leads to radial flushing of liquid metal, giving rise to a ridge around the crater and long filaments along the crater walls. Moreover, in a more external area (up to a distance of about 1 mm from the laser spot center), the surface shows bubbles and long cracks. The results have been compared with similar experiments on W, where the volume of ablated metal was about 10 times lower. This strictly depends on the latent heat of fusion and latent heat of vaporization of W, which are remarkably higher than those of Mo.

The effect of hydrogen on the mechanical properties and microstructure evolution of Ti–45Al–9Nb (at.%) alloy under uniaxial tension at high temperature is investigated in [7]. The constitutive relations among stress, temperature and strain rate in the alloy were determined together with analyses of the microstructure. Due to the presence of hydride $(TiAl)H_x$, the elongation shows a declining trend with increasing strain rate at the same deformation temperature. Here, 0.8 at.% H softened the Ti–45Al–9Nb alloy and reduced the high-temperature plastic deformability. Microstructure examination showed that there are more residual lamellae in the hydrogenated alloy, and the extent of dynamic recrystallization is lower than that of the unhydrogenated alloy. Three types of cracks were also evidenced in the hydrogenated alloy: inter-lamellar, trans-lamellar and along-lamellar colony boundary cracks.

The last paper [8] deals with microstructural characteristics and corrosion behavior of Al–Fe alloys produced by high-frequency induction sintering from a powder mixture of pure Al and variable contents of Fe. The morphology of the produced alloys was investigated by SEM, whereas the crystalline intermetallic phases were determined by XRD. The corrosion behavior of the Al–Fe alloys was studied using the techniques of cyclic polarization (CP) and electrochemical impedance spectroscopy (EIS). It was demonstrated that the addition of Fe into an Al matrix leads to an improvement in the hardness and corrosion resistance of the alloy.

Acknowledgments: As Guest Editors, we would like to especially thank Bunny Zou, Section Managing Editor, for her support and active role in the publication. We are also grateful to the entire staff of the *Coatings* Editorial Office for the collaboration. Furthermore, we are thankful to all of the contributing authors and reviewers; without your excellent work, it would not have been possible to accomplish this Special Issue that we hope will be a piece of interesting reading and reference literature.

Conflicts of Interest: The authors declare no conflict of interest.

References

1. Shivakoti, I.; Kibria, G.; Cep, R.; Pradhan, B.B.; Sharma, A. Laser surface texturing for biomedical applications: A Review. *Coatings* **2021**, *11*, 124. [CrossRef]
2. Bolli, E.; Kaciulis, S.; Mezzi, A. ESCA as a tool for exploration of metals' surface. *Coatings* **2020**, *10*, 1182. [CrossRef]
3. Bolli, E.; Fava, A.; Ferro, P.; Kaciulis, S.; Mezzi, A.; Montanari, R.; Varone, A. Cr segregation and impact fracture in a martensitic stainless steel. *Coatings* **2020**, *10*, 843. [CrossRef]
4. Zhang, C.; Li, P.; Dong, H.; Jin, D.; Huang, J.; Mao, F.; Chen, C. Repetitive impact wear behaviors of the tempered 25Cr3Mo2NiWV Fe-based steel. *Coatings* **2020**, *10*, 107. [CrossRef]
5. Mele, C.; Lionetto, F.; Bozzini, B. An erosion-corrosion investigation of coated steel for applications in the oil and gas field, based on bipolar electrochemistry. *Coatings* **2020**, *10*, 92. [CrossRef]
6. Montanari, R.; Pakhomova, E.; Rossi, R.; Richetta, M.; Varone, A. Surface morphological features of molybdenum irradiated by a single laser pulse. *Coatings* **2020**, *10*, 67. [CrossRef]
7. Yu, Q.; Wen, D.; Wang, S.; Kong, B.; Wu, S.; Xiao, T. Effect of 0.8 at.% H on the mechanical properties and microstructure evolution of a Ti–45Al–9Nb alloy under uniaxial tension at high temperature. *Coatings* **2020**, *10*, 52. [CrossRef]
8. Seikh, A.H.; Baig, M.; Singh, J.K.; Mohammed, J.A.; Luqman, M.; Abdo, H.S.; Khan, A.R.; Alharthi, N.H. Microstructural and corrosion characteristics of Al–Fe alloys produced by high-frequency induction-sintering process. *Coatings* **2019**, *9*, 686. [CrossRef]

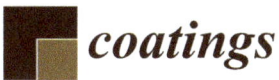

Review

Laser Surface Texturing for Biomedical Applications: A Review

Ishwer Shivakoti [1,*], Golam Kibria [2], Robert Cep [3], Bal Bahadur Pradhan [1] and Ashis Sharma [1]

[1] Department of Mechanical Engineering, Sikkim Manipal Institute of Technology, Sikkim Manipal University, Majhitar, East Sikkim 737136, India; bbpradhan1@reddiffmail.com (B.B.P.); ashz_1974@yahoo.com (A.S.)
[2] Department of Mechanical Engineering, Aliah University, Kolkata 700160, India; prince1983me@gmail.com
[3] VSB-Technical University Ostrava, Faculty of Mechanical Engineering, 17. listopadu 2172/15, 708 00 Ostrava, Czech Republic; robert.cep@vsb.cz
* Correspondence: ishwar.siwa@gmail.com

Abstract: For generating a texture or pattern on a work surface, one of the emerging processes is laser surface texturing (LST). It is an effective method for producing texture on a work surface. Literature shows that various lasers have been applied to generate textures on the surface of work materials. Recently, LST has shown tremendous potential in the field of biomedical applications. Applying the LST process, the efficacy of the biomaterial has been drastically improved. This paper presents an in-depth review of laser surface texturing for biomedical applications. The effect of LST on important biomaterial has been thoroughly studied; it was found that LST has extreme potential for surface modification of biomaterial and can be utilized for biomedical applications.

Keywords: laser micromachining; surface texturing; surface roughness; biomedical engineering; tribology

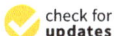

Citation: Shivakoti, I.; Kibria, G.; Cep, R.; Pradhan, B.B.; Sharma, A. Laser Surface Texturing for Biomedical Applications: A Review. *Coatings* **2021**, *11*, 124. https://doi.org/10.3390/coatings11020124

Received: 23 October 2020
Accepted: 18 January 2021
Published: 22 January 2021

Publisher's Note: MDPI stays neutral with regard to jurisdictional claims in published maps and institutional affiliations.

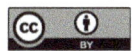

Copyright: © 2021 by the authors. Licensee MDPI, Basel, Switzerland. This article is an open access article distributed under the terms and conditions of the Creative Commons Attribution (CC BY) license (https://creativecommons.org/licenses/by/4.0/).

1. Introduction

Surface texturing is a method of producing a defined pattern or texture on a work surface. It is an effective method of surface alteration for enhancing the tribological properties of the material, such as load capacity, wear resistance and coefficient of friction [1]. The same has been used in magnetic recording sliders [2], mechanical seals [3]. Various texturing processes such as LST, electric discharge texturing, focused ion beams, electrochemical machining, hot embossing, lithography, mechanical texturing has been employed by researchers to generate micro/nanopattern on the work surface. Among all, laser surface texturing (LST) has become a potential texturing method and has been widely used by researchers due to its high-efficiency, excellent controllability, environment friendly, and accuracy. In LST, melting and vaporization of material take place due to ablation when a high-energy beam of laser impinges the work surface. Laser ablation is divided into two types; (i) pyrolytic and (ii) photolytic process. The material absorbs the laser energy, and this energy is converted into heat, and the material starts to melt and vaporize in case of the pyrolytic process. In the photolytic process, absorption of photon induces chemical reaction and overcomes the binding energy of the material [4,5]. The microstructures can act as small traps for debris and behave as micro-reservoir for lubricant which reduces the friction [6]. LST has been successfully applied to various engineering materials like ceramic [7,8], metals [9,10], polymers [11]. This method has been successfully used in various engineering applications in the biomedical, tribology, coating domains. Various patterns/textures have been generated by LST to enhance the tribological behavior of the material. Not only that, but the process also enhances the coefficient of friction and wear resistance of the material. Some of the patterns include dimple and microgroove of various shapes and sizes [12,13]. The paper presents an in-depth review of LST on various applications related to biomedical. In addition, the important achievements obtained by various researchers are discussed in the paper with a critical review and microscopic view of machined surfaces.

2. Methods of Laser Surface Texturing

The literature shows various methods for the generation of textures or patterns produced on the work surface. Among them, widely used methods are texturing using laser ablation and texturing using laser interference. This section presents an in-depth review of laser surface texturing using these methods.

2.1. Texturing Using Laser Ablation

During the laser ablation process, a focused beam of the laser is made to irradiate on the work surface, and it removes the material due to heating, which leads to melt and vaporization of the work material from the irradiated zone. Selective material is removed, and the surface topography is modified [11]. The laser ablation process can remove material in micron-level precision at a faster rate [14] and is an effective technique for developing textures [15]. LST using laser ablation phenomena has been successfully utilized by many researchers. Fabrication of superhydrophobic surface on the gold-coated aluminum plate was successfully generated using the fiber laser ablation process [16]. The kinematic model was also developed to forecast the texture achieved after PLA once the laser impinges to the surface and achieves its use to develop innovative beam paths for the generation of intricate geometrical surfaces [17]. Figure 1 depicts the schematic representation of the laser processing green ceramics. This Nd:YAG laser has a pulse duration of 10 ns and a wavelength of 1064 nm. Using a computer-controlled system, the laser power was controlled through the software interface. Using a scanner, the beam was bent perpendicularly and then; the beam was concentrated using a focusing lens. The laser system has a three-dimensional XYZ stage (precision of the XYZ stage is 10 pm), and for laser texturing, green ZrCb ceramics were placed on this stage. The pattern of laser texture was generated using the computer connected with this laser system.

The laser textured surface results in lower transmittance when compared to the untextured polycarbonate surface using laser ablation [18]. Dimples or pillars were successfully fabricated on the substrate, and diamond-like carbon deposition was done. This leads to improvement of the wear characteristics of the surface [19]. Xing et al. examined the impact of laser parameter on microchannel width, depth and material removal rate while fabricating in PCD using direct laser ablation and laser-induced plasma [20]. Liu et al. fabricated a microtextured groove (30–50 µm width and 15–50 µm depth) on ZrO_2 ceramic. The influence of the laser variable was studied; it has been found that the laser variable has a substantial effect on texture quality [21].

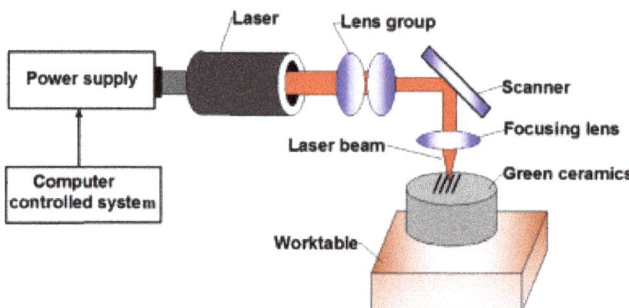

Figure 1. Representational illustration of laser surface texturing of green ceramic [22]. Reprinted from [22]. Copyright from Elsevier 2009.

2.2. Texturing Using Laser Interference

The patterns in this method are fabricated due to interference of two, three or four high-power pulsed laser beams, which permits periodic local heating of work surface by photothermal interaction among laser and work surface [22]. Direct laser interference patterning (DLIP) is a method for creating texture on the technical surfaces [23]. DLIP method are engaged in the development of optical biosensors based on Biophotonic Sensing Cells (BICELLs) [24]. Many studies have been carried out to fabricate a texture/pattern using DLIP [25,26]. Peter et al. developed a DLIP set up on the principle of four beam interference [27]. The group of researchers also shows that the ultrashort pulsed DLIP is a useful method for creating repeated surface structures on steel material and appropriate for retention and adjunct of bacteria [28].

Laser interference lithography has also been utilized for the fabrication of nanoscale patterns on silicon substrates. It has been observed that the consistent dot patterns are obtained in a region of 20 mm (W) and 20 mm (L) with a half-pitch size of nearby 190, 250, and 370 nm by enhancing the power to 0.600 mW/cm^2 [29]. Surface treatment of aluminum has been carried out, and results have revealed that the laser texturing using the two-beam interference method is an effective method for the removal of contamination and surface oxide from the work surface [30]. Furlan et al. fabricated a pattern using DLIP on magnesium alloy and studied laser parameters to understand the relationship between fluence and quality of feature [31]. Morales et al. examined the impact of laser parameter on texture homogeneity during DLIP on Ti–6Al–4V, and the group of researchers found the enhancement of the texture homogeneity by 80–90% [32]. Cardoso et al. fabricated the hierarchical periodic surface on Al2024 alloy using direct laser writing (DLW) and DLIP and found the superhydrophobic surface after one week of fabrication process [33]. Sola et al. processed ophthalmic polydimethylsiloxane PDMS polymers using DLIP and observed damage in photo-based thermal and chemical in the laser-scanned area [34].

3. Laser Surface Texturing for Biomedical Applications

Biocompatibility of a material with host tissues is one of the most thriving areas of research in recent times. Materials with superior biocompatibility are appropriate in applications related to transplantation of tissue and bone [35]. The successful use of gold in a dental implant for centuries shows the use of material for biomedical applications, and the evolvement of biomaterial in the past centuries shows its extensive use in implants. The biomaterials are classified as metallic, ceramic, polymeric, and composite [36]. A texture on the implant can be obtained through grit blasting technique, acid etching, anodic oxidation and chemical vapor deposition. These methods are quick and simple, but the replicability of these methods is inferior. Compared with the above methods, LST is a quick, clean and precise method for implant modification and has been found to be a prospective technique for modification of implant [37,38]. Pereira et al. observed that laser ablation, blended thermal treatment, is a prospective method to produce a hydrophilic surface on ceramic implants by increasing the surface wettability [39]. Cunha et al. showed that the ultrafast LST technique on Ti–6Al–4V increases the surface wettability and regulates the performance of human mesenchymal stem cells (hMSCs) by altering the cytoskeleton shape, FAPs distribution and area, and proliferation [40]. Stango et al. performed coating of hydroxyapatite (HAP) on 316LSS and Ti–6Al–4V implant textured with laser and found that the laser textured surface provides more resistance to corrosion and shows that the surface is suitable for biomedical application [41]. Yu et al. created a microtexture on a titanium surface and concluded that the structured texture enhances the cell adhesion and performs an essential function in contact guidance [42].

3.1. LST on Titanium and Its Alloys for Biomedical Applications

Materials like titanium (and Ti alloys) reveal a high specific strength, low electrical conductivity, corrosion resistance, makes it suitable for dental implantology and in biomedical applications and is used extensively since the early 1970s [43,44]. The reaction among the host tissue and titanium depends on the surface texture of the implant profile [45]. The biomedical applications of titanium alloys include bone plates, artificial hip joints and knee joints, screws used in fixing fractures, pacemakers, cardiac valve prostheses, and artificial hearts [46]. In addition to material, surface topography has a significant effect on the morphology of the cell its orientation, behavior and activity [47]. Though the material possesses outstanding thermo-physical properties and excellent biocompatible, owing to having a high friction coefficient and low wear resistance, the application area of such extraordinary material is limited. To surmount this, the surface treatment of the material is very much essential. Researchers across the globe have adopted many methods for the surface treatment of titanium and its alloys [48]. The laser micro/nanotexturing process modifies the surface properties related to osseointegration, namely biocompatibility, protein adsorption and cell/surface interactions [49]. Shot peening and acid etching and then laser treatment has been employed on Ti material (grade 2) and revealed the change of surface from hydrophobic to hydrophilic, and adsorption of proteins were mostly found in laser textured surface [50]. The researchers found that deposition of biphasic calcium phosphate occurs on textured Ti–6Al–4V materials, and this depicts enhancement in bioactivity, proliferation and cell adhesion and can be possibly utilized for dental and orthopedic related applications [51]. The significance of microgroove width on anti-corrosion and bio-tribological properties was studied during the coating of graphene oxide on Ti–6Al–4V and found improvement in anti-corrosion and antiwear properties [52]. Figure 2 shows the schematic representation of the ultraviolet (UV) solid laser. The wavelength of the UV laser is 355 nm, and the maximum power of the laser is 5 W. The laser is generated at the laser head, and the generated laser beam was passed through two galvanometric mirrors. Using an F-theta scanning lens, the laser beam then transferred to the top surface of the workpiece material. This F-theta lens has been engineered to provide the highest performance in laser scanning or engraving system. The distance between the F-theta lens and workpiece material surface measures the focusing condition during the laser texturing process.

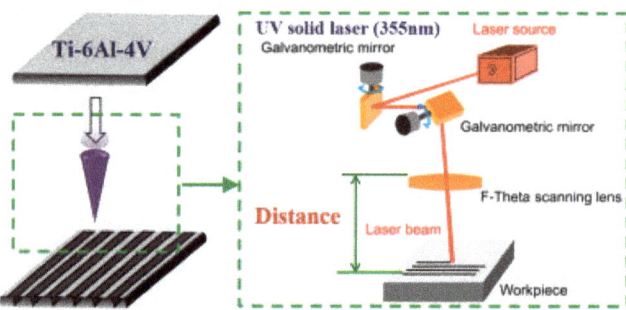

Figure 2. Schematic representation of laser processing of microgroove on Ti–6Al–4V [52]. Reprinted from [52]. Copyright from Elsevier 2020.

The overlay structure generated on titanium alloy enhances the mechanical properties, and further, this process refines the grain of the alloy. Further, the hybrid approach of drenched treatment in m-SBF with textured formation is estimated to be an effective as well as environmentally compatible approach to extend the durability of bone screws and reduces the hurdles of slightly osteoporotic implants [53]. Figure 3 depicts SEM images of the un-textured and textured specimens: (a, a_1) untextured surface, (b, b_1) micro-bulge ring arrays (c, c_1) micro-smooth ring arrays, and (d, d_1) micro-smooth stacked ring. The laser microtexturing effectively reduces the bacteria attachment as compared to abrasive blasted surfaces during LST of Ti–6Al–4V [54]. A group of researchers has synthesized textured bioactive Ca–P coating having 100 and 200 μm placing on Ti–6Al–4V substrate. The authors demonstrated the better cytoskeleton association and propagation of the mouse MC3T3-E1 osteoblast-like cell. Further, improvement in vitro bioactivity and in vitro biocompatibility was achieved in their study [55]. The culture of cells shows that microgrooves on titanium alloy created by LST substantially increase the augmentation and distinction of MC3T3-E1 cells, which indicates the improvement in bioactivity [56].

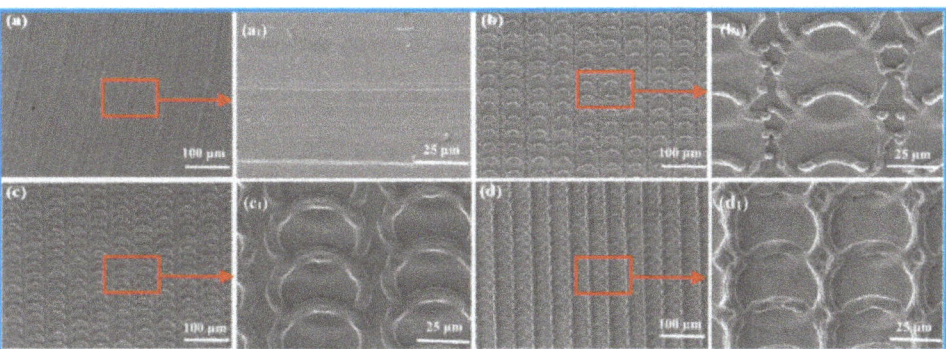

Figure 3. SEM images of the un-textured and textured surfaces: (**a,a₁**) untextured surface, (**b,b₁**) micro-bulge ring arrays (**c,c₁**) micro-smooth ring arrays, and (**d,d₁**) micro smooth stacked ring [53]. Reprinted from [53]. Copyright from Elsevier 2020.

Surface alteration by Nd-YAG laser on titanium alloy was also performed, and it was revealed that the smooth surface could release extra cell adhesion owing to its rise in surface tension and decrease in contact angle [57]. Further, the detachment of the enzyme test verified that maximum cells are affixed to the LTS at 140 J cm^{-2} and lesser to the untreated sample. The optimized parameter of Nd:YAG laser produces a suitable modification on Ti6Al4V alloy. Both SEM and contact angle, along with histopathological assessment, verify that Ti alloy having better chemical and physical properties is obtained and can be used for biomedical implementations [58]. Coathup et al. produced laser texture superhydrophilic Ti-6Al-4V surface having better surface chemistry and topography which significantly endorses osteoblast adhesion in culture. [59]. Textures fabricated with nanosecond pulsed laser and annealing in Ti–6Al–4V show lesser biofilm development on the textured superhydrophobic surface. The suggested approach improves in decreasing the risk of infection related to implants devoid of using cytotoxic bactericidal agents [60]. Borcherding et al. fabricated a texture on titanium alloy with titanium dioxide coating [61]. The experimental findings showed the improvement in cell feasibility on textured surfaces related to pure titanium, suggesting good cytocompatibility. Figure 4 illustrates the SEM image of human osteoblast-like cells, picturing the sticking on a time of three days at various surface conditions. Texturing like dimple structures was generated on the titanium alloy [62]. This textured surface exhibits substantial progress in bioactivity with respect to the $Ca_3(PO4)_2$ depositing rate in Hank's solution. The cell proliferation (XTT) result shows analogous cell feasibility of textured Ti–6Al–4V compared to un-textured Ti-alloy. Laser texturing using femtosecond laser was carried out to reduce the establishment of Grade 2 titanium alloy surface by *Staphylococcus aureus* and the successive biofilm creation [63]. The process decreases bacterial adhesion and biofilm formation related to the polished surface. The authors also concluded that femtosecond LST is a capable way for bestowing orthopedic and dental implants with antibacterial characteristics and reducing implant-related infections. Ultrafast LST has been applied as a method for surface modification of Ti–6Al–4V dental and orthopedic implant to enhance osteoblastic assurance of human mesenchymal stem cells (hMSCs) [64]. The authors concluded that nanotextures involving laser-irradiated regular surface configurations and nano-sized pillars are capable of enhancing hMSC discrimination into an osteoblastic lineage. Three distinct topographies were processed with femtosecond laser at various laser parameters, and it was shown to enhance osteogenesis and hinder the adipogenesis of MSCs [65]. The formed nano-ripples only supported the osteoblastic commitment. Furthermore, the combination of nano-ripples and micro-patterns (pits) improved osteogenic ability. Raimbault et al. investigated the biological operation impacts of laser (femtosecond) formed structure on performance of cell and concluded that cells are responsive to the nanostructure excepting that the microstructure size is deeper than 5 µm and near to the cell size [66]. Cells are responsive to the microscale structure spreads with respect to these structures.

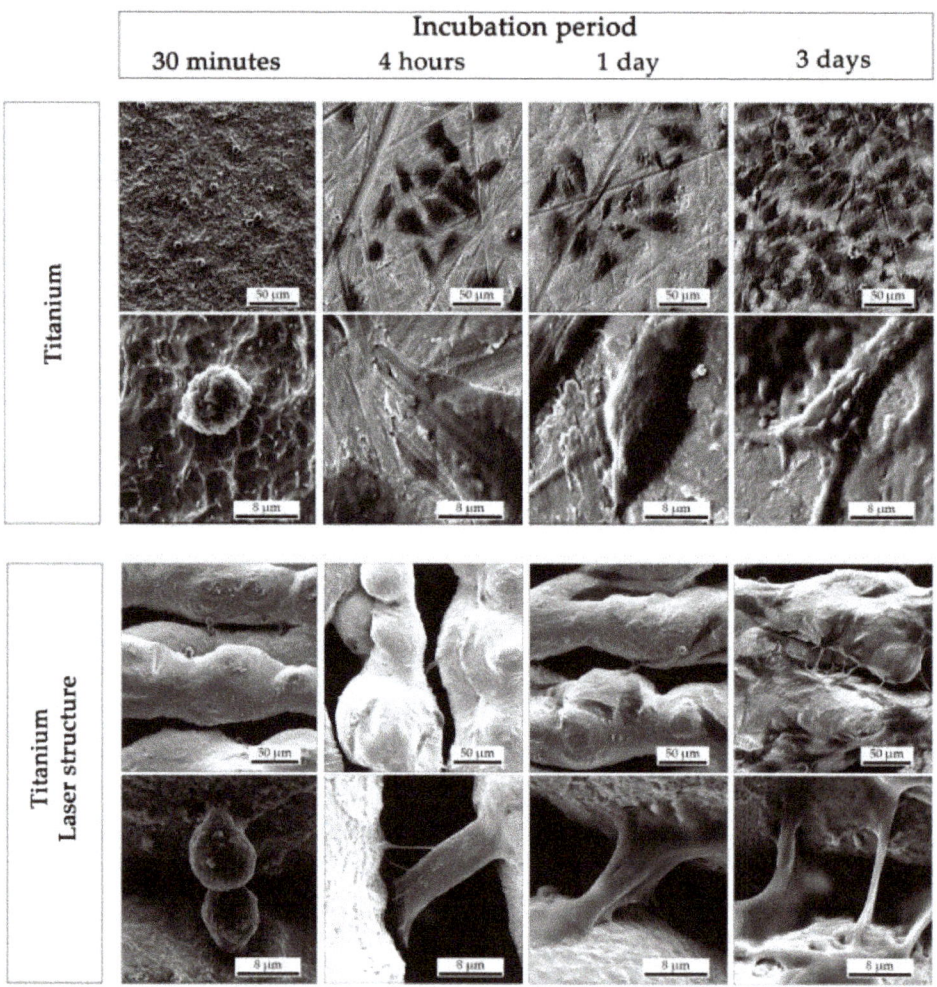

Figure 4. *Cont.*

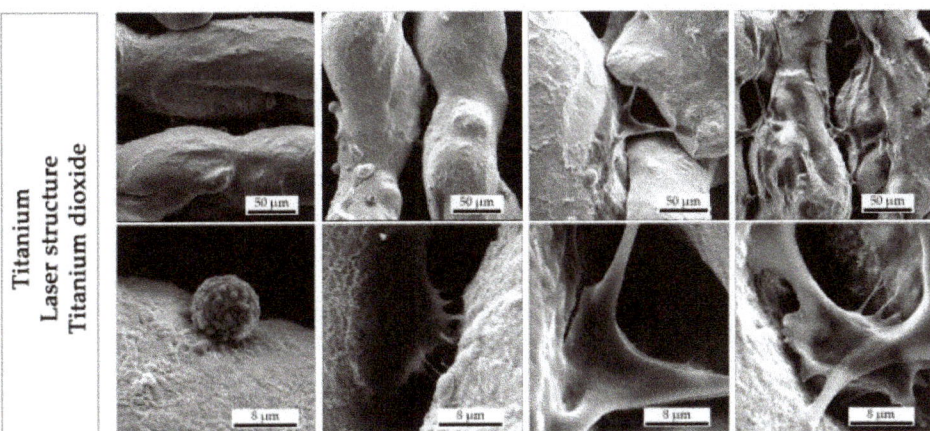

Figure 4. SEM image of human osteoblast-like cells (MG-63), picturing the adhesion on a time of three days at various surface conditions [61].

3.2. LST on Zirconia for Biomedical Application

Zirconia dental implants have appeared as an alternative to titanium implants due to their capability to osseointegrate, excellent mechanical properties, enhanced biocompatibility. They also possess other useful properties like its transparency and white color, which imitates the natural teeth [67,68]. Moura et al. presented LST on zirconia implant and shows that textured surface has greater chemical affinity among bone and 3Y-TZP disks, and thus, the process promotes better bone imprisonment on the surface [69]. The friction test of laser-treated and subsequent deposition of a HAp-coated zirconia reveals superb adhesion of HAp coating on textured zirconia surface. In addition, the bioactive coating reliability does not concede through implant insertion [70]. Figure 5 illustrates the SEM images of HAp-coated zirconia textured surface after the friction tests against bone and the subsequent EDS spectra of evident zones, Z1 and Z2.

The combined effect of laser texturing and cold-pressing methods on zirconia exhibits an effective method for fabrication of zirconia implants with tailored surface designs corresponding to the properties essential for specific application [71]. Guimarães et al. show that microtexture on zirconia surfaces coated by 45S5 BG and HAp glass via a dip coating. Subsequently, the biologically active coating remained laser sintered and revealed that square texture (groove width of 100 µm) functionality with a biologically active coating represents an increase in 90% of cell feasibility related to flat surfaces following incubation of 48 h [72]. Figure 6 illustrates the SEM images of the as-sintered (AS) and flat surface, indicating the common and detailed view of cells propagating. Madeira et al. fabricated Aunps and Agµps-functionalized zirconia produced by spray deposition, laser adhesion and laser texturing, additive laser strategies, respectively shows nice performance to friction test suggesting that the integrity is not influenced through implant attachment [73]. The laser processing method may be effectively used for the formation of specifically structured thin films on ceramic material and their biopolymer composites and bulk zirconia material, which improves mechanical and biological response in dental implants [74]. Utilizing Nd:YAG laser, the surface texture was formed to enhance the mechanical interlocking of hydroxyapatite (HAp) powder and subsequently enhances its adhesion to zirconia [75]. The outcomes depict that it is likely to create texture by altering energy density and atmosphere. Moreover, a good quantity of retained and sintered bioactive material was retrieved with higher laser power and lower scanning speed. Figure 7 depicts SEM images of the HAp sintered within the textured at various laser power and scan speeds.

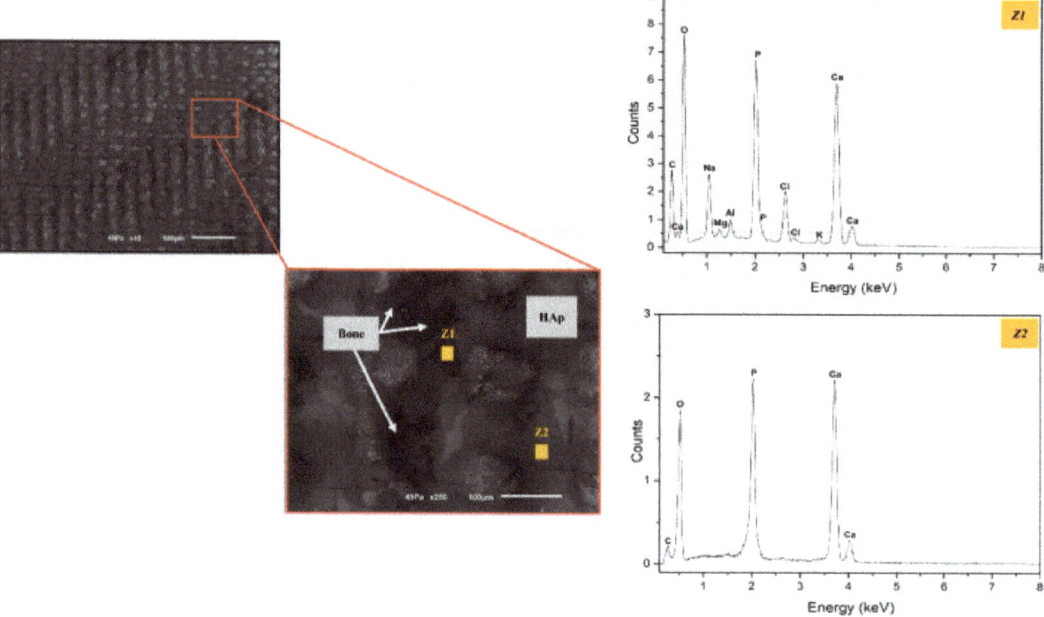

Figure 5. SEM images of HAp-coated zirconia textured surface, after the friction tests against bone and the subsequent EDS spectra of evident zones, Z1 and Z2 [70]. Reprinted from [70]. Copyright from Elsevier 2020.

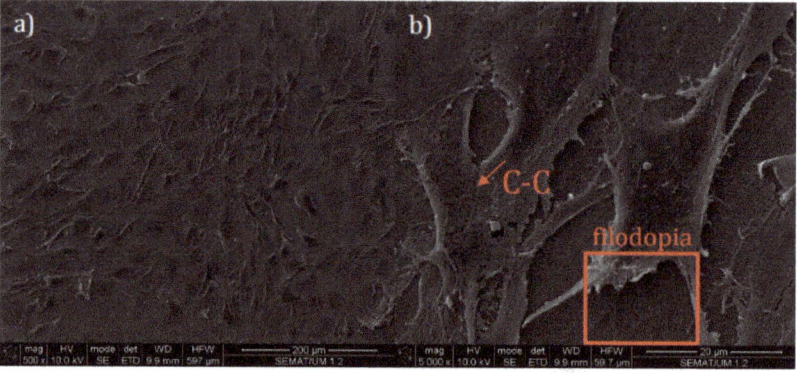

Figure 6. SEM images of the as-sintered (AS) and flat surface, indicating the (**a**) general and (**b**) detailed view of cells spreading [72]. Reprinted from [72]. Copyright from Elsevier 2020.

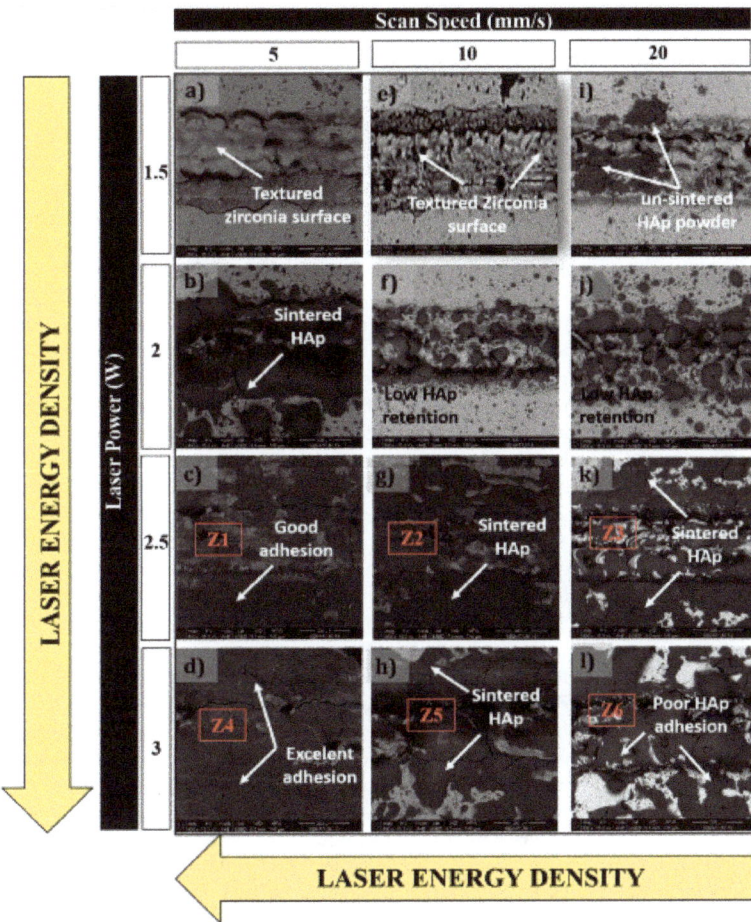

Figure 7. SEM images of the hydroxyapatite (HAp) sintered within the textured at various laser power and scan speeds [75]. Reprinted from [75]. Copyright from Elsevier 2018.

Delgado-Ruı́z et al. studied the appropriateness of femtosecond laser for micro texturing cylindrical zirconia dental implants surface [76]. Sixty-six zirconia implants were utilized and split into three groups: as a surface with no laser treatment, micro-grooved texture and micro-grooved texture. The result shows that femtosecond laser micro texturing extends an attractive option to traditional surface treatments of zirconia implants due to its precision and lesser damage on surrounding regions. A study of the femtosecond laser ablation method was done to develop micro and nano-level structures to alter the surface topography of alumina-toughened zirconia (ATZ) [77]. The treated surface shows suggestively high expression of osteogenic transcription factors, genes. In addition, the development of a mineralized extracellular matrix was observed compared to the untreated surface. The linear microgroove arrays and superimposed crossline microgroove textured in zirconia substrates depicts that for steep surfaces, parallel micro line surfaces are capable of handling cell growth only, but the curved ones decrease the initial response and depict the least osteogenic response [78].

3.3. LST on Polymer

Polymers are natural or synthetic substances composed of very large molecules. These are developed by connecting a huge number of units known as monomers. In the area of biomedical applications, these polymers are extensively used [14]. The laser ablation of PTFE films of several thickness and densities has shown that laser treatment of polymer-tissue will be helpful in clinical tool [79]. The use of various laser wavelengths (1.064 µm, 532 nm and 355 nm) on the carbon-coated surface of polyethylene (UHMWPE) materials and the effect of laser parameters on material surface properties depicts that the 355 nm and 532 nm wavelength laser results in comparatively suitable for improving the surface conditions such as wettability and surface roughness of UHMWPE. The outcomes were revealed for maximizing surface conditions, and these also significantly affect the interaction process between cell and material [80]. CO_2 laser texturing of poly (L-lactide) presents the capability to adjust the physical and structural characteristics of the material's surface to the needs of the cells with substantial alterations in the mechanical properties of the treated polymer surface [81]. Study of laser variable on the wettability, roughness and hardness of polypropylene material was carried out using 1.064 µm, 355 nm and 532 nm lasers. The authors suggested that laser wavelengths are appropriate for increasing the surface roughness of polypropylene [82]. The Ra values are more than 1 µm, and this value is a minimum essential value to enhance the bonding of bone in the implant surface as per the literature. Mirzadeh et al. improved the hydrophilicity and biocompatibility of ethylene-propylene rubber N-vinylpyrrolidone (NVP) and 2-hydroxyethyl methacrylate (HEMA) by grafting to the polymer using pulsed CO_2 laser at various laser power. Alveolar macrophages cultured on un-treated films shows the greater attachment of cell with good propagating and flattening while supports adhere to the treated EPR showed round with marginal cytoplasmic spreading and ruffling [83]. Using excimer lasers, Dinca P et al. carried out experimentation for single-step creation on natural composite substrates for roughness gradients and concluded that cell behavior of engineered polymer might participate a vital function for the progress of the next-generation of bioactive interfaces for perusing cell integration [84]. Koufaki et al. investigated the cell adhesion, and possibility on high rough polymeric surfaces with gradient roughness ratio and wettability formulated by laser micro/nano-textured Si surfaces shows that superior adhesion of both cell types was observed in microstructured surfaces linked to the unstructured surface. Furthermore, PC12 cells were noticed to adhere nicely to the patterned surface [85]. Direct laser writing on the biodegradable polymer to produce microchannels for attachment of C2C12 myoblast cells in the microchannels depicts a high degree of alignment after four days as cell proliferated into a merging patch inside the channels [86]. Waugh et al. presented the surface characteristics and properties of nylon 6,6 treated by CO_2 laser and suggested that laser textured surfaces enhance the biomimetic properties of nylon 6,6 in terms of osteoblast cell response [87].

3.4. LST on Other Material for Biomedical Application

Magnesium (Mg) alloys have drawn great interest for use as implants. Hu et al. modified the Mg–6Gd–0.6Ca alloy with laser for investigating the cell behavior for the same and concluded that MC3T3-E1 exhibits better sticking to the laser-treated surface [88]. The LT method efficiently enhances the bactericidal properties of copper surfaces, and the LT-Cu kills bacteria selectively; no cytotoxicity was noted compared to mammalian cells [89]. Qin et al. have used laser surface texturing to create three types of texture on Co–Cr–Mo alloys surfaces and concluded that textured Co–Cr–Mo surface influence osteoblast proliferation, gene expression and morphology [90]. Purnama et al. fabricated a texture on SS316L and explored the impacts of the textured material on the proliferation of adhesion and endothelial cell arrangement. The finding shows that the textured surfaces supported these three processes of cells [91]. The texturing of AISI 304 steel at various laser fluences enables the fabrication of surface microfluidic appliances for chemical and biomedical applications [92].

4. Summary

The paper presents an in-depth review of laser surface texturing for biomedical applications. The researcher has used various types of lasers, such as carbon-dioxide laser, excimer laser, fiber laser, etc., to produce texture to explore the efficacy of the process and its impact on proliferation, osseointegration, cell adhesion, etc. The widely used biomaterial such as titanium and its alloy and zirconia has been reviewed thoroughly, indicating important contributions achieved and representation of suitable micrographs and plots. Apart from these materials, other material that has been used for biomedical applications also has been studied in-depth, mentioning the striking contributions of the research and development in the field of LST.

(i) Though there are many studies on titanium and its alloys and zirconia for biomedical applications, very limited work has been carried out considering the effect of laser parameters on the laser texturing process. The parametric analysis of several surface properties (like roughness, wettability, hardness, etc.) is essential for the overall improvement of the process and commercial application in the emerging area;

(ii) For other material, more research needs to be carried out for exploring the physics in LST, and clinical trials must be carried out to confirm the feasibility for its application in the biomedical domain. Further, it was observed that laser surface texturing has become a potential method for surface modification of biomaterial and may be successfully utilized for biomedical applications.

Author Contributions: Conceptualization, I.S., G.K.; methodology, B.B.P., R.C.; validation, A.S., I.S., R.C., I.S., G.K.; resources, G.K., I.S.; writing—I.S., G.K. All authors have read and agreed to the published version of the manuscript.

Funding: This research was funded by TMA Pai, Sikkim Manipal University.

Institutional Review Board Statement: Not applicable.

Informed Consent Statement: Not applicable.

Conflicts of Interest: The authors declare no conflict of interest.

References

1. Bhaduria, D.; Batala, A.; Dimova, S.S.; Zhangb, Z.; Dongb, H.; Fallqvistc, M.; M'Saoubid, R. On design and tribological behaviour of laser textured surfaces. *Procedia CIRP* **2017**, *60*, 20–25. [CrossRef]
2. Hausmann, U.P.; Joerges, P.; Heinzl, J.; Talke, F.E. Nano-texturing of magnetic recording sliders via laser ablation. *Microsyst. Technol.* **2009**, *15*, 1747–1751. [CrossRef]
3. Etsion, I.; Halperin, G. A laser surface textured hydrostatic mechanical seal. *Tribol. Trans.* **2002**, *45*, 430–434. [CrossRef]
4. Mao, B.; Arpith Siddaiah, Y.L.; Pradeep, L.M. Laser surface texturing and related techniques for enhancing tribological performance of engineering materials: A review. *J. Manuf. Process.* **2020**, *53*, 153–173. [CrossRef]
5. Arslan, A.; Masjuki, H.H.; Kalam, M.A.; Varman, M.; Mufti, R.A.; Mosarof, M.H.; Khuong, L.S.; Quazi, M.M. Surface texture manufacturing techniques and tribological effect of surface texturing on cutting tool performance: A review. *Crit. Rev. Solid State Mater. Sci.* **2016**, *41*, 447–481. [CrossRef]
6. Joshi, B.; Tripathi, K.; Gyawali, G.; Lee, S.W. The effect of laser surface texturing on the tribological performance of different Sialon ceramic phases. *Prog. Nat. Sci. Mater. Int.* **2016**, *26*, 415–421. [CrossRef]
7. Li, D.; Chen, X.; Guo, C.; Tao, J.; Tian, C.; Deng, Y.; Zhang, W. Micro surface texturing of alumina ceramic with nanosecond laser. *Procedia Eng.* **2017**, *174*, 370–376. [CrossRef]
8. Xing, Y.; Deng, J.; Feng, X.; Yu, S. Effect of laser surface texturing on Si3N4/TiC ceramic sliding against steel under dry friction. *Mater. Design (1980–2015)* **2013**, *52*, 34–45. [CrossRef]
9. Šugár, P.; Šugárová, J.; Frnčík, M. Laser surface texturing of tool steel: Textured surfaces quality evaluation. *Open Eng.* **2016**, *6*, 90–97. [CrossRef]
10. Tripathi, K.; Gyawali, G.; Joshi, B.; Amanov, A.; Wohn, S. Improved tribological behavior of grey cast Iron Under low and high viscous lubricants by laser surface texturing. *Mater. Perform. Charact.* **2017**, *6*, 24–41. [CrossRef]
11. Riveiro, A.; Maçon, A.L.; del Val, J.; Comesaña, R.; Pou, J. Laser surface texturing of polymers for biomedical applications. *Front. Phys.* **2018**, *6*, 16. [CrossRef]
12. Ezhilmaran, V.; Vasa, N.J.; Vijayaraghavan, L. Investigation on generation of laser assisted dimples on piston ring surface and influence of dimple parameters on friction. *Surf. Coat. Technol.* **2018**, *335*, 314–326. [CrossRef]

13. Liang, L.; Yuan, J.; Li, X.; Yang, F.; Jiang, L. Wear behavior of the micro-grooved texture on WC-Ni3Al cermet prepared by laser surface texturing. *Int. J. Refract. Met. Hard Mater.* **2018**, *72*, 211–222. [CrossRef]
14. White, N.; Eder, K.; Byrnes, J.; Cairney, J.M.; McCarroll, I.E. Laser ablation sample preparation for atom probe tomography and transmission electron microscopy. *Ultramicroscopy* **2020**, *220*, 113161. [CrossRef]
15. Shum, P.W.; Zhou, Z.F.; Li, K.Y. To increase the hydrophobicity and wear resistance of diamond-like carbon coatings by surface texturing using laser ablation process. *Thin Solid Film.* **2013**, *544*, 472–476. [CrossRef]
16. Eskandari, M.J.; Shafyei, A.; Karimzadeh, F. Investigation of wetting properties of gold nanolayer coated aluminum surfaces textured with continuous-wave fiber laser ablation. *Thin Solid Film.* **2020**, *711*, 138278. [CrossRef]
17. Kong, M.C.; Miron, C.B.; Axinte, D.A.; Davies, S.; Kell, J. On the relationship between the dynamics of the power density and workpiece surface texture in pulsed laser ablation. *CIRP Ann.* **2012**, *61*, 203–206. [CrossRef]
18. Yilbas, B.S.; Khaled, M.; Abu-Dheir, N.; Al-Aqeeli, N.; Said, S.A.; Ahmed, A.O.; Varanasi, K.K.; Toumi, Y.K. Wetting and other physical characteristics of polycarbonate surface textured using laser ablation. *Appl. Surf. Sci.* **2014**, *320*, 21–29. [CrossRef]
19. Shum, P.W.; Zhou, Z.F.; Li, K.Y. To increase the hydrophobicity, non-stickiness and wear resistance of DLC surface by surface texturing using a laser ablation process. *Tribol. Int.* **2014**, *78*, 1–6. [CrossRef]
20. Xing, Y.; Zhang, K.; Huang, P.; Liu, L.; Wu, Z. Assessment machining of micro-channel textures on PCD by laser-induced plasma and ultra-short pulsed laser ablation. *Opt. Laser Technol.* **2020**, *125*, 106057. [CrossRef]
21. Liu, Y.; Liu, L.; Deng, J.; Meng, R.; Zou, X.; Wu, F. Fabrication of micro-scale textured grooves on green ZrO2 ceramics by pulsed laser ablation. *Ceram. Int.* **2017**, *43*, 6519–6531. [CrossRef]
22. Zabila, Y.; Perzanowski, M.; Dobrowolska, A.; Kac, M.; Polit, A.; Marszalek, M. Direct laser interference patterning: Theory and application. *Acta Phys. Pol. Ser. A Gen. Phys.* **2009**, *115*, 591. [CrossRef]
23. Rosenkranz, A.; Hans, M.; Gachot, C.; Thome, A.; Bonk, S.; Mücklich, F. Direct laser interference patterning: Tailoring of contact area for frictional and antibacterial properties. *Lubricants* **2016**, *4*, 2. [CrossRef]
24. Sanza, F.J.; Langheinrich, D.; Berger, J.; Hernandez, A.L.; Dani, S.; Casquel, R.; Lavin, A.; Otón, A.; Santamaría, B.; Laguna, M.; et al. Direct laser interference patterning (DLIP) technique applied to the development of optical biosensors based on biophotonic sensing cells (bicells). *Int. Soc. Opt. Photonics* **2015**, *9351*, 935114.
25. El-Khoury, M.; Alamri, S.; Voisiat, B.; Kunze, T.; Lasagni, A.F. Fabrication of hierarchical surface textures using multi-pulse direct laser interference patterning with nanosecond pulses. *Mater. Lett.* **2020**, *258*, 126743. [CrossRef]
26. Baumann, R.; Milles, S.; Leupolt, B.; Kleber, S.; Dahms, J.; Lasagni, A.F. Tailored wetting of copper using precise nanosecond direct laser interference patterning. *Opt. Lasers Eng.* **2020**, *137*, 106364. [CrossRef]
27. Peter, A.; Onuseit, V.; Freitag, C.; Faas, S.; Graf, T. Flexible, compact and picosecond laser capable four-beam interference setup. In Proceedings of the Lasers in Manufacturing Conference, Munich, Germany, 18–22 June 2017; pp. 1–8.
28. Peter, A.; Lutey, A.H.; Faas, S.; Romoli, L.; Onuseit, V.; Graf, T. Direct laser interference patterning of stainless steel by ultrashort pulses for antibacterial surfaces. *Opt. Laser Technol.* **2020**, *123*, 105954. [CrossRef]
29. Choi, J.; Chung, M.H.; Dong, K.Y.; Park, E.M.; Ham, D.J.; Park, Y.; Song, I.S.; Pak, J.J.; Ju, B.K. Investigation on fabrication of nanoscale patterns using laser interference lithography. *J. Nanosci. Nanotechnol.* **2011**, *11*, 778–781. [CrossRef]
30. Chen, J.; Sabau, A.S.; Jones, J.F.; Hackett, A.C.; Daniel, C.; Warren, D. Aluminum surface texturing by means of laser interference metallurgy. In *Light Metals*; Springer: Cham, Switzerland, 2015; pp. 427–429.
31. Furlan, V.; Biondi, M.; Demir, A.G.; Pariani, G.; Bianco, A.; Previtali, B. Direct laser texturing using two-beam interference patterning on biodegradable magnesium alloy. In Proceedings of the International Congress on Applications of Lasers & Electro-Optics, San Diego, CA, USA, 16–20 October 2016; p. 182.
32. Aguilar-Morales, A.I.; Alamri, S.; Kunze, T.; Lasagni, A.F. Influence of processing parameters on surface texture homogeneity using Direct Laser Interference Patterning. *Opt. Laser Technol.* **2018**, *107*, 216–227. [CrossRef]
33. Cardoso, J.T.; Aguilar-Morales, A.I.; Alamri, S.; Huerta-Murillo, D.; Cordovilla, F.; Lasagni, A.F.; Ocaña, J.L. Superhydrophobicity on hierarchical periodic surface structures fabricated via direct laser writing and direct laser interference patterning on an aluminium alloy. *Opt. Lasers Eng.* **2018**, *111*, 193–200. [CrossRef]
34. Sola, D.; Lavieja, C.; Orera, A.; Clemente, M.J. Direct laser interference patterning of ophthalmic polydimethylsiloxane (PDMS) polymers. *Opt. Lasers Eng.* **2018**, *106*, 139–146. [CrossRef]
35. Radmanesh, M.; Kiani, A. Effects of laser pulse numbers on surface biocompatibility of titanium for implant fabrication. *J. Biomater. Nanobiotechnol.* **2015**, *6*, 168. [CrossRef]
36. Kurella, A.; Dahotre, N.B. Surface modification for bioimplants: The role of laser surface engineering. *J. Biomater. Appl.* **2005**, *20*, 5–50. [CrossRef] [PubMed]
37. Yu, Z.; Yin, S.; Zhang, W.; Jiang, X.; Hu, J. Picosecond laser texturing on titanium alloy for biomedical implants in cell proliferation and vascularization. *J. Biomed. Mater. Res. Part B Appl. Biomater.* **2020**, *108*, 1494–1504. [CrossRef]
38. Fiorucci, M.P.; López, A.J.; Ramil, A. Surface modification of Ti6Al4V by nanosecond laser ablation for biomedical applications. *J. Phys. Conf. Ser.* **2015**, *605*, 012022. [CrossRef]
39. Pereira, R.S.; Moura, C.G.; Henriques, B.; Chevalier, J.; Silva, F.S.; Fredel, M.C. Influence of laser texturing on surface features, mechanical properties and low-temperature degradation behavior of 3Y-TZP. *Ceram. Int.* **2020**, *46*, 3502–3512. [CrossRef]

40. Cunha, A.; Oliveira, V.; Serro, A.P.; Zouani, O.E.; Almeida, A.; Durrieu, M.C.; Vilar, R. Ultrafast laser texturing of Ti-6Al-4V surfaces for biomedical applications. In Proceedings of the International Congress on Applications of Lasers & Electro-Optics, Miami, FL, USA, 6–10 October 2013; pp. 910–918.
41. Stango, S.A.; Karthick, D.; Swaroop, S.; Mudali, U.K.; Vijayalakshmi, U. Development of hydroxyapatite coatings on laser textured 316 LSS and Ti-6Al-4V and its electrochemical behavior in SBF solution for orthopedic applications. *Ceram. Int.* **2018**, *44*, 3149–3160. [CrossRef]
42. Yu, Z.; Yang, G.; Zhang, W.; Hu, J. Investigating the effect of picosecond laser texturing on microstructure and biofunctionalization of titanium alloy. *J. Mater. Process. Technol.* **2018**, *255*, 129–136. [CrossRef]
43. Sidambe, A.T. Biocompatibility of advanced manufactured titanium implants—A review. *Materials* **2014**, *7*, 8168–8188. [CrossRef]
44. Schiff, N.; Grosgogeat, B.; Lissac, M.; Dalard, F. Influence of fluoride content and pH on the corrosion resistance of titanium and its alloys. *Biomaterials* **2002**, *23*, 1995–2002. [CrossRef]
45. Pou, P.; Riveiro, A.; del Val, J.; Comesaña, R.; Penide, J.; Arias-González, F.; Soto, R.; Lusquiños, F.; Pou, J. Laser surface texturing of Titanium for bioengineering applications. *Procedia Manuf.* **2017**, *13*, 694–701. [CrossRef]
46. Elias, C.N.; Lima, J.H.; Valiev, R.; Meyers, M.A. Biomedical applications of titanium and its alloys. *Jom* **2008**, *60*, 46–49. [CrossRef]
47. Tiainen, L.; Abreu, P.; Buciumeanu, M.; Silva, F.; Gasik, M.; Guerrero, R.S.; Carvalho, O. Novel laser surface texturing for improved primary stability of titanium implants. *J. Mech. Behav. Biomed. Mater.* **2019**, *98*, 26–39. [CrossRef]
48. Ramskogler, C.; Warchomicka, F.; Mostofi, S.; Weinberg, A.; Sommitsch, C. Innovative surface modification of Ti6Al4V alloy by electron beam technique for biomedical application. *Mater. Sci. Eng. C* **2017**, *78*, 105–113. [CrossRef]
49. Shukla, P.; Waugh, D.G.; Lawrence, J.; Vilar, R. Laser surface structuring of ceramics, metals and polymers for biomedical applications: A review. In *Laser Surface Modification of Biomaterials*; Woodhead Publishing: Cambridge, UK, 2016; pp. 281–299.
50. Kuczyńska, D.; Kwaśniak, P.; Marczak, J.; Bonarski, J.; Smolik, J.; Garbacz, H. Laser surface treatment and the resultant hierarchical topography of Ti grade 2 for biomedical application. *Appl. Surf. Sci.* **2016**, *390*, 560–569. [CrossRef]
51. Behera, R.R.; Das, A.; Hasan, A.; Pamu, D.; Pandey, L.M.; Sankar, M.R. Deposition of biphasic calcium phosphate film on laser surface textured Ti-6Al-4V and its effect on different biological properties for orthopedic applications. *J. Alloy. Compd.* **2020**, *842*, 155683. [CrossRef]
52. Wang, C.; Li, Z.; Zhao, H.; Zhang, G.; Ren, T.; Zhang, Y. Enhanced anticorrosion and antiwear properties of Ti-6Al-4V alloys with laser texture and graphene oxide coatings. *Tribol. Int.* **2020**, *152*, 106475. [CrossRef]
53. Xu, Y.; Liu, W.; Zhang, G.; Li, Z.; Hu, H.; Wang, C.; Zeng, X.; Zhao, S.; Zhang, Y.; Ren, T. Friction stability and cellular behaviors on laser textured Ti-6Al-4V alloy implants with bioinspired micro-overlapping structures. *J. Mech. Behav. Biomed. Mater.* **2020**, *109*, 103823. [CrossRef]
54. Uhlmann, E.; Schweitzer, L.; Kieburg, H.; Spielvogel, A.; Huth-Herms, K. The Effects of Laser Microtexturing of Biomedical Grade 5 Ti-6Al-4V Dental Implants (Abutment) on Biofilm Formation. *Procedia CIRP* **2018**, *68*, 184–189. [CrossRef]
55. Paital, S.R.; Bunce, N.; Nandwana, P.; Honrao, C.; Nag, S.; He, W.; Banerjee, R.; Dahotre, N.B. Laser surface modification for synthesis of textured bioactive and biocompatible Ca-P coatings on Ti-6Al-4V. *J. Mater. Sci. Mater. Med.* **2011**, *22*, 1393–1406. [CrossRef]
56. Zheng, Q.; Mao, L.; Shi, Y.; Fu, W.; Hu, Y. Biocompatibility of Ti-6Al-4V titanium alloy implants with laser microgrooved surfaces. *Mater. Technol.* **2020**, 1–10. [CrossRef]
57. Khosroshahi, M.E.; Mahmoodi, M.; Saeedinasab, H.; Tahriri, M. Evaluation of mechanical and electrochemical properties of laser surface modified Ti-6Al-4V for biomedical applications: In vitro study. *Surf. Eng.* **2008**, *24*, 209–218. [CrossRef]
58. Khosroshahi, M.E.; Tavakoli, J.; Mahmoodi, M. Analysis of bioadhesivity of osteoblast cells on titanium alloy surface modified by Nd: YAG laser. *J. Adhes.* **2007**, *83*, 151–172. [CrossRef]
59. Coathup, M.J.; Blunn, G.W.; Mirhosseini, N.; Erskine, K.; Liu, Z.; Garrod, D.R.; Li, L. Controlled laser texturing of titanium results in reliable osteointegration. *J. Orthop. Res.* **2017**, *35*, 820. [CrossRef]
60. Patil, D.; Aravindan, S.; Kaushal Wasson, M.; Rao, P.V. Fast fabrication of superhydrophobic titanium alloy as antibacterial surface using nanosecond laser texturing. *J. Micro Nano-Manuf.* **2018**, *6*, 011002. [CrossRef]
61. Borcherding, K.; Marx, D.; Gätjen, L.; Specht, U.; Salz, D.; Thiel, K.; Wildemann, B.; Grunwald, I. Impact of Laser Structuring on Medical-Grade Titanium: Surface Characterization and In Vitro Evaluation of Osteoblast Attachment. *Materials* **2020**, *13*, 2000. [CrossRef]
62. Kumari, R.; Scharnweber, T.; Pfleging, W.; Besser, H.; Majumdar, J.D. Laser Surface Textured Titanium Alloy (Ti-6Al-4V)-Part II-Studies on Bio-compatibity. *Appl. Surf. Sci.* **2015**, *357*, 750–758. [CrossRef]
63. Cunha, A.; Elie, A.M.; Plawinski, L.; Serro, A.P.; do Rego, A.M.; Almeida, A.; Urdaci, M.C.; Durrieu, M.C.; Vilar, R. Femtosecond laser surface texturing of titanium as a method to reduce the adhesion of Staphylococcus aureus and biofilm formation. *Appl. Surf. Sci.* **2016**, *360*, 485–493. [CrossRef]
64. Cunha, A.; Zouani, O.F.; Plawinski, L.; Botelho do Rego, A.M.; Almeida, A.; Vilar, R.; Durrieu, M.C. Human mesenchymal stem cell behavior on femtosecond laser-textured Ti-6Al-4V surfaces. *Nanomedicine* **2015**, *10*, 725–739. [CrossRef]
65. Dumas, V.; Guignandon, A.; Vico, L.; Mauclair, C.; Zapata, X.; Linossier, M.T.; Bouleftour, W.; Granier, J.; Peyroche, S.; Dumas, J.C.; et al. Femtosecond laser nano/micro patterning of titanium influences mesenchymal stem cell adhesion and commitment. *Biomed. Mater.* **2015**, *10*, 055002. [CrossRef]

66. Raimbault, O.; Benayoun, S.; Anselme, K.; Mauclair, C.; Bourgade, T.; Kietzig, A.M.; Girard-Lauriault, P.L.; Valette, S.; Donnet, C. The effects of femtosecond laser-textured Ti-6Al-4V on wettability and cell response. *Mater. Sci. Eng. C* **2016**, *69*, 311–320. [CrossRef]
67. Apratim, A.; Eachempati, P.; Salian, K.K.; Singh, V.; Chhabra, S.; Shah, S. Zirconia in dental implantology: A review. *J. Int. Soc. Prev. Community Dent.* **2015**, *5*, 147. [CrossRef]
68. Depprich, R.; Zipprich, H.; Ommerborn, M.; Naujoks, C.; Wiesmann, H.P.; Kiattavorncharoen, S.; Lauer, H.C.; Meyer, U.; Kübler, N.R.; Handschel, J. Osseointegration of zirconia implants compared with titanium: An in vivo study. *Head Face Med.* **2008**, *4*, 30. [CrossRef]
69. Moura, C.G.; Pereira, R.; Buciumeanu, M.; Carvalho, O.; Bartolomeu, F.; Nascimento, R.; Silva, F.S. Effect of laser surface texturing on primary stability and surface properties of zirconia implants. *Ceram. Int.* **2017**, *43*, 15227–15236. [CrossRef]
70. Faria, D.; Henriques, B.; Souza, A.C.; Silva, F.S.; Carvalho, O. Laser-assisted production of HAp-coated zirconia structured surfaces for biomedical applications. *J. Mech. Behav. Biomed. Mater.* **2020**, *112*, 104049. [CrossRef]
71. Faria, D.; Madeira, S.; Buciumeanu, M.; Silva, F.S.; Carvalho, O. Novel laser textured surface designs for improved zirconia implants performance. *Mater. Sci. Eng. C* **2020**, *108*, 110390. [CrossRef]
72. Mesquita-Guimarães, J.; Detsch, R.; Souza, A.C.; Henriques, B.; Silva, F.S.; Boccaccini, A.R.; Carvalho, O. Cell adhesion evaluation of laser-sintered HAp and 45S5 bioactive glass coatings on micro-textured zirconia surfaces using MC3T3-E1 osteoblast-like cells. *Mater. Sci. Eng. C* **2020**, *1091*, 10492. [CrossRef]
73. Madeira, S.; Barbosa, A.; Moura, C.G.; Buciumeanu, M.; Silva, F.S.; Carvalho, O. Aunps and Agμps-functionalized zirconia surfaces by hybrid laser technology for dental implants. *Ceram. Int.* **2020**, *46*, 7109–7121. [CrossRef]
74. Daskalova, A.; Angelova, L.; Carvalho, A.; Trifonov, A.; Nathala, C.; Monteiro, F.; Buchvarov, I. Effect of surface modification by femtosecond laser on zirconia based ceramics for screening of cell-surface interaction. *Appl. Surf. Sci.* **2020**, *26*, 145914. [CrossRef]
75. Carvalho, O.; Sousa, F.; Madeira, S.; Silva, F.S.; Miranda, G. HAp-functionalized zirconia surfaces via hybrid laser process for dental applications. *Opt. Laser Technol.* **2018**, *106*, 157–167. [CrossRef]
76. Delgado-Ruíz, R.A.; Calvo-Guirado, J.L.; Moreno, P.; Guardia, J.; Gomez-Moreno, G.; Mate-Sánchez, J.E.; Ramirez-Fernández, P.; Chiva, F. Femtosecond laser microstructuring of zirconia dental implants. *J. Biomed. Mater. Res. Part B Appl. Biomater.* **2011**, *96*, 91–100. [CrossRef] [PubMed]
77. Carvalho, A.; Cangueiro, L.; Oliveira, V.; Vilar, R.; Fernandes, M.H.; Monteiro, F.J. Femtosecond laser microstructured Alumina toughened Zirconia: A new strategy to improve osteogenic differentiation of hMSCs. *Appl. Surf. Sci.* **2018**, *435*, 1237–1245. [CrossRef]
78. Elena Sima, L.; Bonciu, A.; Baciu, M.; Anghel, I.; Dumitrescu, L.N.; Rusen, L.; Dinca, V. Bioinstructive Micro-Nanotextured Zirconia Ceramic Interfaces for Guiding and Stimulating an Osteogenic Response In Vitro. *Nanomaterials* **2020**, *10*, 2465. [CrossRef] [PubMed]
79. Makropoulou, M.; Serafetinides, A.A.; Skordoulis, C.D. Ultra-violet and infra-red laser ablation studies of biocompatible polymers. *Lasers Med Sci.* **1995**, *10*, 201–206. [CrossRef]
80. Riveiro, A.; Soto, R.; Del Val, J.; Comesaña, R.; Boutinguiza, M.; Quintero, F.; Lusquiños, F.; Pou, J. Laser surface modification of ultra-high-molecular-weight polyethylene (UHMWPE) for biomedical applications. *Appl. Surf. Sci.* **2014**, *302*, 236–242. [CrossRef]
81. Tomanik, M.; Kobielarz, M.; Filipiak, J.; Szymonowicz, M.; Rusak, A.; Mroczkowska, K.; Antończak, A.; Pezowicz, C. Laser Texturing as a Way of Influencing the Micromechanical and Biological Properties of the Poly (L-Lactide) Surface. *Materials* **2020**, *13*, 3786. [CrossRef]
82. Riveiro, A.; Soto, R.; Del Val, J.; Comesaña, R.; Boutinguiza, M.; Quintero, F.; Lusquiños, F.; Pou, J. Texturing of polypropylene (PP) with nanosecond lasers. *Appl. Surf. Sci.* **2016**, *374*, 379–386. [CrossRef]
83. Mirzadeh, H.; Katbab, A.A.; Burford, R.P. CO2-laser graft copolymerization of HEMA and NVP onto ethylene-propylene rubber (EPR) as biomaterial-(III). *Radiat. Phys. Chem.* **1995**, *46*, 859–862. [CrossRef]
84. Dinca, V.; Alloncle, P.; Delaporte, P.; Ion, V.; Rusen, L.; Filipescu, M.; Mustaciosu, C.; Luculescu, C.; Dinescu, M. Excimer laser texturing of natural composite polymer surfaces for studying cell-to-substrate specific response. *Appl. Surf. Sci.* **2015**, *352*, 82–90. [CrossRef]
85. Koufaki, N.; Ranella, A.; Aifantis, K.E.; Barberoglou, M.; Psycharakis, S.; Fotakis, C.; Stratakis, E. Controlling cell adhesion via replication of laser micro/nano-textured surfaces on polymers. *Biofabrication* **2011**, *3*, 045004. [CrossRef]
86. Yeong, W.Y.; Yu, H.; Lim, K.P.; Ng, K.L.; Boey, Y.C.; Subbu, V.S.; Tan, L.P. Multiscale topological guidance for cell alignment via direct laser writing on biodegradable polymer. *Tissue Eng. Part C Methods* **2010**, *16*, 1011–1021. [CrossRef] [PubMed]
87. Waugh, D.; Lawrence, J. Laser surface processing of polymers for biomedical applications. In *Laser-Assisted Fabrication of Materials*; Springer: Berlin/Heidelberg, Germany, 2013; pp. 275–318.
88. Hu, G.; Guan, N; Lu, L.; Zhang, J.; Lu, N., Guan, Y. Engineered functional surfaces by laser microprocessing for biomedical applications. *Engineering* **2018**, *4*, 822–830. [CrossRef]
89. Selvamani, V.; Zareei, A.; Elkashif, A.; Maruthamuthu, M.K.; Chittiboyina, S.; Delisi, D.; Li, Z.; Cai, L.; Pol, V.G.; Seleem, M.N.; et al. Hierarchical micro/mesoporous copper structure with enhanced antimicrobial property via laser surface texturing. *Adv. Mater. Interfaces* **2020**, *7*, 1901890. [CrossRef]
90. Qin, L.; Zeng, Q.; Wang, W.; Zhang, Y.; Dong, G. Response of MC3T3-E1 osteoblast cells to the microenvironment produced on Co–Cr–Mo alloy using laser surface texturing. *J. Mater. Sci.* **2014**, *49*, 2662–2671. [CrossRef]

91. Purnama, A.; Furlan, V.; Dessi, D.; Demir, A.G.; Tolouei, R.; Paternoster, C.; Levesque, L.; Previtali, B.; Mantovani, D. Laser surface texturing of SS316L for enhanced adhesion of HUVECs. *Surf. Eng.* **2018**, 1–10. [CrossRef]
92. Krylach, I.V.; Kudryashov, S.I.; Olekhnovich, R.O.; Moskvin, M.K.; Uspenskaya, M.V. Tuning water wetting angle of a steel surface via nanosecond laser ablative nano/microtexturing for chemical and biomedical microfluidic applications. *Laser Phys. Lett.* **2019**, *16*, 105602. [CrossRef]

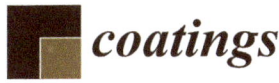 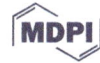

Review

ESCA as a Tool for Exploration of Metals' Surface

Eleonora Bolli [1,2,*], **Saulius Kaciulis** [2] **and Alessio Mezzi** [2]

1. Department of Industrial Engineering, University of Rome "Tor Vergata", Via del Politectico 1, 00133 Rome, Italy
2. Institute for the Study of Nanostructured Materials, ISMN—CNR, Monterotondo Stazione, 00015 Rome, Italy; Saulius.kaciulis@cnr.it (S.K.); alessio.mezzi@cnr.it (A.M.)
* Correspondence: Eleonora.bolli@ismn.cnr.it; Tel.: +39-06-90672892

Received: 29 October 2020; Accepted: 30 November 2020; Published: 3 December 2020

Abstract: The main principles and development of electron spectroscopy for chemical analysis (ESCA) are briefly reviewed. The role of ESCA techniques (X-ray photoelectron spectroscopy and Auger electron spectroscopy) in the investigation of metallic surfaces is discussed, evidencing their importance and analytical potentiality. An overview is given of a series of recent experimental cases of ESCA application for the characterization of different metals and metallic alloys, illustrating the main results and various phenomena, such as the formation of impurity defects, corrosion, migration of constituent elements in various alloys, clustering in liquid alloy, etc., that can occur on the surface and the interface of investigated materials. These materials comprise the collection coins of noble metals, some metal alloys and Ni-based superalloys, nitride coatings on stainless steel, composite material with TiAlV alloy, treated austenitic steels, and graphene interface with polycrystalline metal foils. The present review could be particularly recommended for the newcomers to the research field of surface analysis and its application for various metals, their treatments, and possible modifications in operating conditions.

Keywords: surface analysis; metals and alloys; metal coatings; XPS; AES; SPEM

1. Introduction

From the very beginning of surface science around 1960, coinciding with the discovery of electron spectroscopy for chemical analysis (ESCA) [1], a great part of the first surface analysis studies has been dedicated to various metals [2]. This is easily understandable because the metals are stable in ultrahigh vacuum (UHV), and their surface is relatively clean (or can be easily cleaned) and is not modified under soft X-rays or electron beam. Therefore, during the initial boom of surface analysis—namely when the main experimental techniques were developed, the main principles were established, and spectroscopic catalogues were created—great attention of this research was given to the surface of metals, and in particular, the transition metals and noble ones. In this period, new scientific journals dedicated to surface analysis were also born, such as *Journal of Electron Spectroscopy* and *Related Phenomena*, etc. Classical examples of metals' surface studies can be found already in the first volume of the first journal mentioned [3,4]. Even later, when surface analysis became a common tool in the labs of materials characterization and when the ESCA handbooks of all chemical elements were available [5,6], the application for the surface of metals remained an important research field, as it was emphasized in the first text books on surface analysis [7,8].

Currently, when a great variety of surface-sensitive electron spectroscopies (see [9]) are available everywhere in the world, the most used ones remain X-ray photoelectron spectroscopy (XPS) and Auger electron spectroscopy (AES) that were born with a common term of ESCA. Of course, at present time, surface analyses are aimed at more sophisticated materials than elemental metals, but even for elemental metals these techniques are widely used for the simple and reliable control of surface purity in the fields of materials research and technological applications. It is namely for these reasons that we decided to prepare a short review, illustrating the importance and analytical capabilities of surface analysis for the exploration of metals, including also their modifications induced by operating conditions. In this review, we present the most interesting cases of experimental research carried out in our lab during the last few decades. These cases comprise the surface defects on noble metals (collection coins), some metal alloys and superalloys, nitride coatings on steel, composite material with TiAlV alloy, treatments of austenitic steel, and graphene growth on polycrystalline metals. The common denominator of all these cases is the application of ESCA, i.e., XPS and AES techniques, for materials' characterization.

The main working equations of ESCA are very simple, and they are based on the principle of energy conservation. In the case of XPS, this equation is

$$BE = h\nu - KE - WF, \qquad (1)$$

where BE is the binding energy of the elemental core level, hν is the photon energy of X-rays, KE is the kinetic energy of the emitted photoelectron, and WF is the work function of the spectrometer.

In Auger effect, the electrons from three different atomic levels are involved, resulting in the finally excited Auger electron with kinetic energy equal to the following:

$$KE = EL1 - EL2 - EL3 - WF, \qquad (2)$$

where KE is the kinetic energy of emitted Auger electron; EL1 is the binding energy of the first atomic level, where the hole is created (by X-rays or electron beam); EL2 is the energy of the second level from which the electron is falling down to the lower level EL1; and EL3 is the energy of the third atomic level from which the Auger electron is ejected. Of course, in some chemical elements the last two levels of the Auger process can be located in the valence band, where a core–valence–valence (CVV) Auger peak is then observed. Typical examples of such elements with broad Auger CVV peaks are carbon and silicon. A schematic diagram of the final state in photoemission and Auger excitations is illustrated in Figure 1.

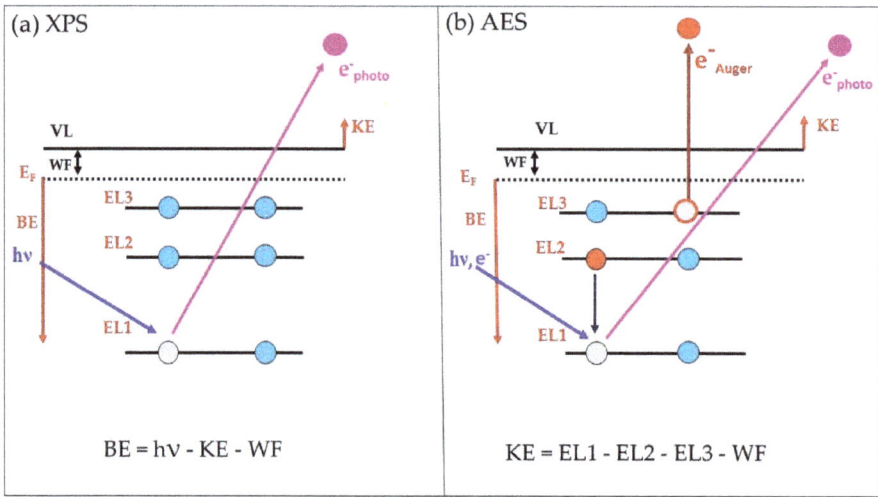

Figure 1. Schematic diagram of the final state in photoemission (**a**) and Auger (**b**) excitations.

From the photoemission and/or Auger spectra, it is possible to identify the chemical elements because the energy of these peaks is characteristic for every element. In the case of superposition of some peaks from different elements, other peaks of the same elements can be used for identification. In most cases, the XPS also permits the chemical state of constituent elements to be identified due to the chemical shift of the photoemission peaks [10]. Both the techniques are surface sensitive because their information depth is limited by the mean free path of the electrons in the solid, which depends on kinetic energy and is typically from 1 to about 10 nm. The detailed description of XPS and AES techniques can be found in numerous text books (e.g., [7–9]) and even online (e.g., [11]).

In the case of AES, the primary electron beam can be easily focused as with electron microscopy, and therefore it is possible not only to achieve a high lateral resolution in spectroscopy but also to acquire the chemical maps of the surface. This mode of operating is called Auger scanning microscopy (SAM). The first two generations of XPS spectrometers were equipped with standard soft X-ray sources (typically with Al and Mg anodes); because of this, the focusing of X-rays was impossible, and the lateral resolution of these instruments was limited to about 0.1–1 mm. Later on, with the introduction of monochromatized X-ray sources and electromagnetic input lenses, the lateral resolution of XPS was improved to about 1–3 microns, allowing also for the operation in XPS imaging mode, i.e., to acquire the surface chemical maps [12,13]. However, quite often this resolution can be too low for the investigation of the submicrometric features or patterns on the sample surface. A much higher lateral resolution of photoemission spectroscopy and imaging can be achieved by using the dedicated beamlines of synchrotron radiation. This technique, which is called scanning photoelectron microscopy (SPEM), enables us to investigate the surface chemical composition at a lateral resolution of about 100 nm [14,15]. It was successfully employed also for some of our experimental cases by using an ESCA microscopy beamline at the synchrotron Elettra in Trieste, Italy. The main features of XPS, AES, and SPEM techniques are summarized in the Table 1, including also the benefits and weak points of their practical applications.

Table 1. Comparison of the main features of three ESCA techniques.

Features	XPS	AES	SPEM
Probe	Soft X-rays	Electrons	Soft X-rays
Spectroscopic signal	Photoelectrons, Auger electrons	Auger electrons	Photoelectrons, Auger electrons
Detectable elements	Li and higher	Li and higher	Li and higher
Sampling depth	0.5–10 nm	0.5–10 nm	0.5–10 nm
Detection limit	1×10^{-4}	1×10^{-3}	1×10^{-4}
Information	Elemental, chemical	Elemental	Elemental, chemical
Quantification	OK	semi	OK
Lateral resolution	>3 µm	>30 nm	>50 nm
Advantages	Chemical bonding, no sample damage	High resolution of chemical imaging	Chemical bonding, chemical imaging
Disadvantages	Poor lateral resolution	Sample charging, beam-induced damage	Beam-induced damage

2. Experimental Techniques

Two different spectrometers were used for the XPS characterization of investigated materials: an aged Escalab MkII (VG Scientific Ltd., East Grinstead, UK) and a modern one, Escalab 250Xi (Thermo Fisher Scientific Ltd., East Grinstead, UK). In both the instruments, the spectroscopy was carried out by concentric hemispherical analyzers operating in a constant pass energy (20 or 40 eV) mode. The first one was equipped with a double-anode (Al/Mg Kα) X-ray source and electrostatic input lens, collecting the signal from the sample area of about 10 mm (large-area mode) and variable to about 0.3 mm (small-area mode). The photoemission signals were registered by a 5-channeltron detector.

The second apparatus was equipped with a monochromatized Al Kα source and a combined system of electrostatic/electromagnetic input lenses. In the spectroscopy mode, this system allowed the diameter of analyzed sample area to vary from 900 to 20 μm, and the photoemission signals were registered by a 6-channeltron detector. In the imaging XPS mode, the best lateral resolution of chemical maps was of about 3 μm, and the signals were registered by a multichannel plate with 128 channels. The charging of insulating samples was suppressed by using a combination of two neutralizing floods: low energy electrons from an in-lens gun and low energy Ar+ ions from an external gun. For the sample surface cleaning and XPS depth profiling in both the Escalabs, rastered Ar+ ion guns were used, i.e., the EX05 model in MkII and the EX06 in 250Xi. The base UHV pressure in the analysis chambers of both spectrometers was always kept below 10^{-9} mbar.

The experiments of AES/SAM were carried out by using a LEG200 electron gun installed on the analysis chamber of Escalab MkII. This excitation source provided the primary beam of electrons with an energy up to 10 keV and a minimum beam diameter of 200 nm. For all the samples, the current of electron beam was kept very low (4–10 nA) in order to avoid any sample surface damage by the electron beam. Seeking to increase the signal-to-noise ratio, all the Auger spectra and chemical maps were acquired in a constant retard ratio (1:2) mode of the analyzer.

All experimental data were processed by the software Avantage v.5 (Thermo Fisher Scientific Ltd.). The peak fitting of photoemission spectra was performed by using the Shirley background, a Voigt peak-shape (mixed Gaussian-Lorentzian with variable ratio), and linked full widths at half maximum (FWHMs) for the same core level. Final calibration of the BE scale was done by fixing the main component of C 1s peak (aliphatic carbon) at 285.0 eV and controlling it, if the Fermi level in the valence band is positioned at BE = 0.0 eV.

High resolution SPEM experiments were performed at the ESCA microscopy beamline of the Elettra synchrotron [14,15]. By using Fresnel zone plate optics, the X-ray beam from the synchrotron source was focused to a microprobe with a diameter of about 150 nm on the sample, which was raster-scanned with respect to the microprobe. Photoelectrons were collected by the SPECS-PHOIBOS 100 hemispherical analyzer and registered by a 48-channel electron detector. All the samples were investigated in both imaging and spectroscopy modes with a 0.2 eV energy resolution by using 500–700 eV photon energy. The overall lateral resolution was below 50 nm. Before the measurements, the samples were cleaned by Ar$^+$ ion sputtering at 2.0 keV energy. After the acquisition, the chemical maps were processed by the Igor v.6.3 software.

3. Experimental Cases of Different Materials

3.1. "Gold Corrosion" in Collection Coins

Can "gold corrosion" occur in gold coins? This question arose approximately two decades ago, when some owners of precious coins unexpectedly found the appearance of numerous stains on their gold coins. After many studies, even using the Pourbaix diagram, this enigma was successfully disclosed because of the application of surface analysis techniques. The chemical composition of these defects was determined, and their source was established.

The study of surface analysis was performed on gold and silver collection coins supplied by the Kunsthistorisches Museum in Vienna (historical Austrian Ducat) and Austrian Mint (coins and their blanks). XPS, AES, and SAM techniques were combined to get qualitative and quantitative information about the surface defects. Their stains, analysed by a stereomicroscope, were generally composed by a dark central area surrounded by a larger outer area, whose colour varied from red to dark blue [16]. The chemical composition of every single stain was determined by XPS. All elements in the spot were quickly identified by the assignment of the peaks found in the survey scan spectrum (Figure 2), whereas their chemical state and atomic concentration were determined by processing the resolved spectra of the main peaks presented in Figure 3 [17].

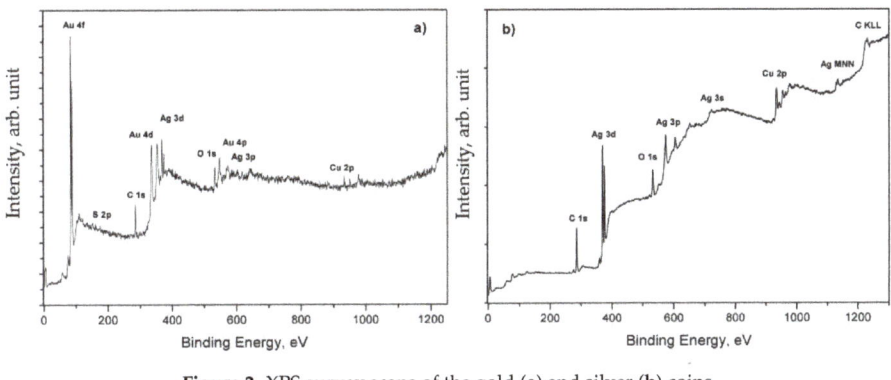

Figure 2. XPS survey scans of the gold (**a**) and silver (**b**) coins.

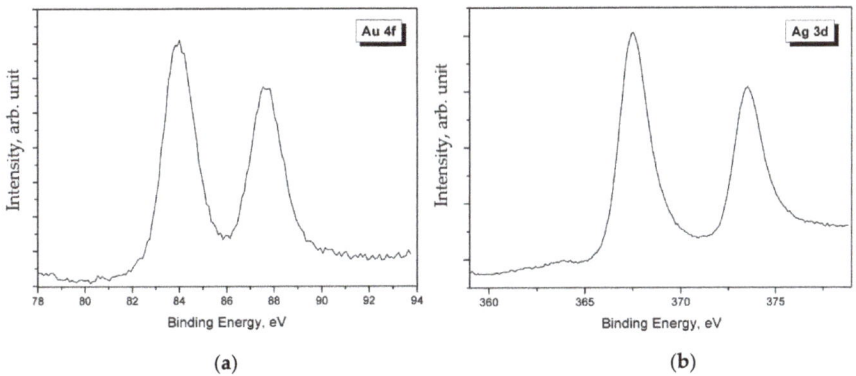

Figure 3. High-resolution XPS spectra of Au 4f (**a**) and Ag 3d (**b**).

The obtained results promptly evidenced a strange composition of the stains on a pure (999.9) gold coin: A contamination with Ag and S was revealed. This was an astonishing finding for a pure gold coin, giving rise to the following questions: how and when had these impurities been added? The obtained results were confirmed by the multipoint AES analysis and SAM chemical maps acquired with a higher lateral resolution of approximately 200 nm, which are presented in Figure 4.

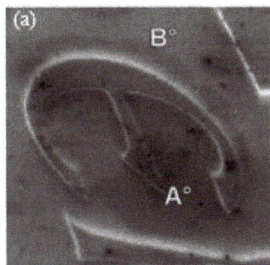 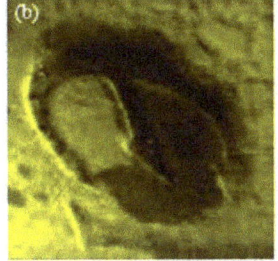 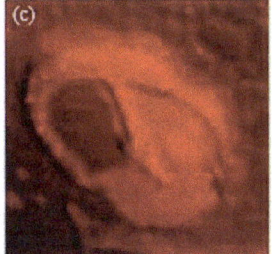

Figure 4. *Cont.*

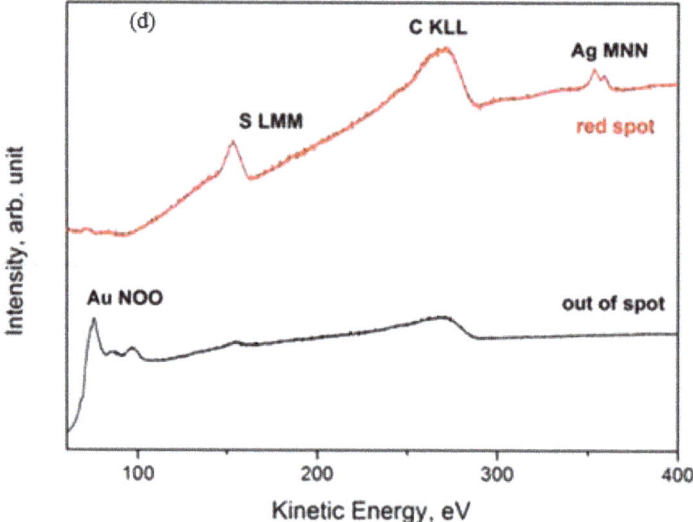

Figure 4. Auger electron spectroscopy (AES) investigation of the defect on gold coin: SEM image—size 1.8 × 1.8 mm² (**a**); Au NOO image (**b**); Ag MNN image (**c**) and AES spectra (**d**) acquired in the red spot (point A) and out of the spot (point B) [17].

The analysis of Ag 3d, Ag LMM, and S 2p spectra gave some indications on their chemical state. As it can be seen in Figure 4, the Ag 3d spectrum was characterized by the typical doublet of the spin-orbit splitting of the core level 3d (Ag $3d_{5/2}$–Ag $3d_{3/2}$), separated by 6.0 eV. The main Ag $3d_{5/2}$ peak was positioned at BE = 368.0 eV. However, it is well known that the Ag 3d signal is one of the few cases where the chemical shift is almost absent, i.e., it is impossible to identify the chemical state of Ag only from photoemission spectra. In these cases, it is necessary to calculate the modified Auger parameter α' by using a very simple formula: α' = BE (Ag $3d_{5/2}$) + KE (Ag LMM) [18]. The value of the Auger parameter can indicate the chemical state (metal, oxide, etc.) of the investigated element. In this case, it was α' = 725.2 – 725.3 eV, which is the typical value for Ag^+ in the silver sulfides, specifically in Ag_2S [5]. The analysis of the S 2p signal confirmed the presence of sulfides, since the S $2p_{3/2}$ peak was positioned at BE = 161.6–161.9 eV [5].

It is interesting to note that the XPS quantitative analysis identified four different scenarios, depending on the color of the spot, which are summarized in Figure 5: (1) grey stains—with Ag, O and S; (2) dark spots—with Ag, O, and S, but also with Au and Cu; (3) red spots—like the grey spots, but with different atomic concentration of the elements; and (4) clean surface—with Au, Cu, and a small amount of O.

Then, the different chemical composition of the stains was investigated by XPS depth profiling, which revealed the different thicknesses of the stains: from 5 to 6 nm for red ones to about 300 nm for dark blackish colored ones. Therefore, the variation of the color was principally related to a different thickness of contamination layer, where the thickness of Ag_2S was always limited to the first 3–5 nm and the second sublayer of metallic Ag continued in depth. These results suggest that a thin, almost transparent, overlayer of sulphide was formed by the interaction of metallic Ag with the sulfur-containing contaminants in air (like H_2S), whereas some bigger silver particles were mechanically embedded into the coin surface during the milling, rolling, or punching of the gold strips.

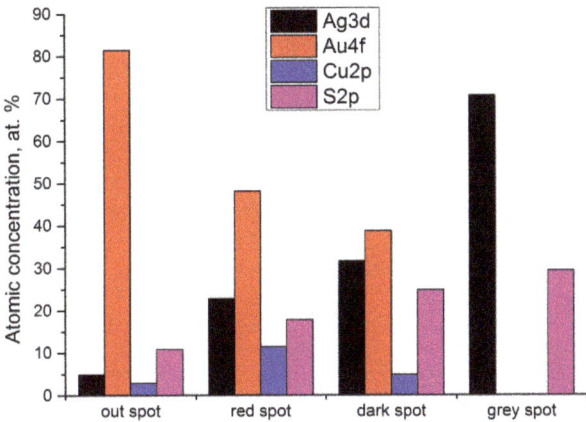

Figure 5. XPS elemental quantification of the different spots on the gold coin.

3.2. Hard Coatings of Nitrides

Hard coatings, based on transition metal nitrides or carbides, are characterized by excellent mechanical properties, suited for steel protection and fabrication of cutting tools. Their performance is continuously improved by the optimization of the fabrication processes, the development of new deposition technologies, and the production of composite materials with enhanced physical and chemical properties. An important contribution to the development of these coatings can be given by the use of surface analysis, which enables us to find the best production conditions and to improve their quality. In this section, the results obtained by the XPS and AES investigations of the TiN-Ti composite and a multilayer CrN–Cr coating are presented. As it can be seen in Figure 6, the deconvolution of the Ti 2p spectrum shows the presence of multiple contributions due to the different chemical states of Ti: the components 3 and 4 located at BE = 458.5 and 456.5 eV were assigned to the chemical states of Ti^{4+} and Ti^{3+} bound to oxygen; the component 1 positioned at BE = 454.1 eV was related to metallic Ti (0); finally, the component 2 positioned at BE = 455.0 eV was assigned to the bonds of Ti–N and Ti–C [19,20].

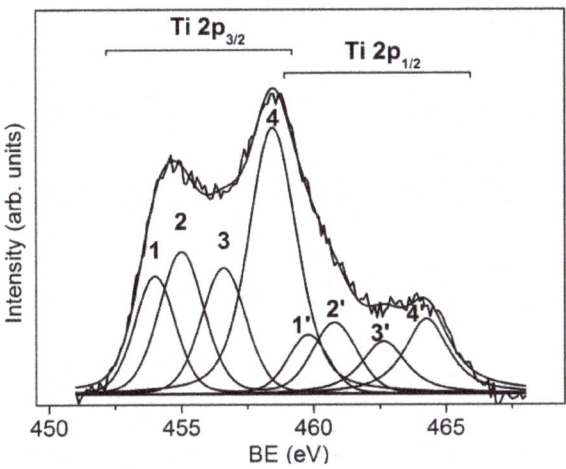

Figure 6. Ti 2p peak fitting of the Ti/TiN composite coating [19].

Naturally, the presence of oxides was caused by the oxidation of metallic Ti in air. After ion sputtering, they were almost removed as it is shown in Figure 7. Of course, the possible influence of the preferential sputtering of oxygen [21,22] to the reduction of oxides cannot be excluded, but in our case this effect was not considered, as this study aimed to determine the composition in the volume of Ti nitride after removal of the native oxides overlayer. By using XPS depth profiling, i.e., alternating cycles of ion sputtering and spectra acquisition, it is possible to investigate the changes of chemical composition until a depth of about 1 µm. From the depth profile shown in Figure 8, it is possible to observe how the content of oxides decreases in depth, whereas the contents of metallic Ti and nitrides increase. This trend was also confirmed by the depth profile of the N 1s signal, which was composed of two peaks positioned at BE = 397.0 and 399.5 eV and was assigned to the bonds of N–Ti and N–O in oxynitride compounds, most probably formed due to environmental contamination. The atomic ratio Ti/N = 3.5 was constant along the depth profiling. This excess of Ti content indicated the formation of composite TiN-Ti.

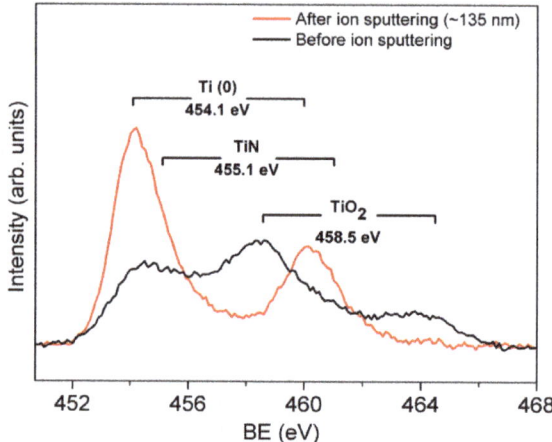

Figure 7. Comparison of the Ti2p signals acquired before and after Ar$^+$ ion sputtering [19].

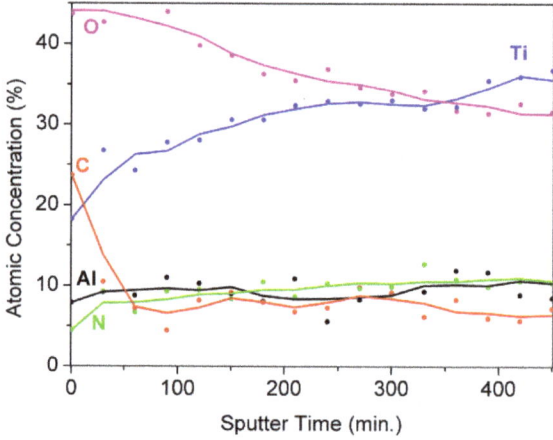

Figure 8. XPS depth profile of the Ti/TiN composite coating. The average sputtering rate was equal to 0.3 nm·min^{-1} [19].

Due to the limited depth of XPS depth profiling, the study of the multilayer coating CrN/Cr/CrN with the thicknesses of 1.5/1.0/1.5 µm was carried out only for the top layer of this coating [23]. In this layer, the signal of Cr 2p (Figure 9) was composed of a typical Cr $2p_{3/2}$–$2p_{1/2}$ doublet, which was positioned at BE = 574.2 eV, and a large peak due to the contribution of multiplet splitting, centered at BE = 576.0 eV. The deconvolution of the N 1s spectrum evidenced the presence of two chemical species: chromium nitride at BE = 397.1 eV and a component of oxynitrides at BE = 398.6 eV, probably due to the presence of a low amount of oxygen in the deposition chamber. The obtained BE values of N 1s and Cr $2p_{3/2}$ (single component) indicated the formation of CrN, excluding the phase of Cr_2N characterized by a noticeably higher value of BE [5]. This supposition was confirmed also by the determined atomic ratio of Cr/N nearly at 1.0. The XPS depth profile, depicted in Figure 10, showed that after removal of the surface contamination, the composition of CrN coating remained almost constant. Since the total thickness of the coating (~4 µm) was too high for XPS depth profiling until the substrate, it was stopped after the removal of ~100 nm of CrN, and the cross section of the coating was further investigated. Due to the limited lateral resolution of XPS, the interfaces of CrN/Cr, Cr/CrN, and CrN/substrate were investigated by the AES/SAM technique.

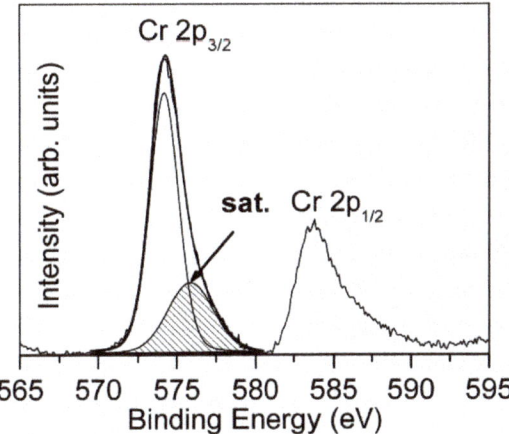

Figure 9. Peak fitting of Cr 2p spectrum acquired on the top of the multilayer coating [23].

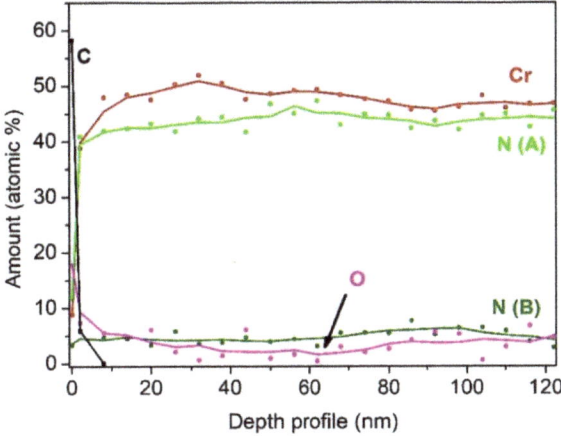

Figure 10. XPS depth profile of the first CrN layer in composite coating. The average sputtering rate was equal to 0.3 nm·min^{-1} [23].

Figure 11 shows the SEM image and the multipoint AES analyses carried out on the cross section of the sample. The AES spectra were acquired on different points, moving from the substrate (region 1) to the top of the coating (region 4). The substrate was characterized by the presence of Fe LMM peaks (KE = 594.0, 652.0 and 705.7 eV) and the low-intensity KLL peaks of C and O (see Figure 11b). In Regions 2 and 4, the peaks of Cr $L_3M_{23}M_{45}$ (KE = 530.6 eV) and N KLL (KE = 385.4 eV) were registered, whereas in Region 3, only a peak of Cr $L_3M_{23}M_{45}$ was present. In addition, the chemical maps were acquired by SAM, where the investigated area of the sample was represented by pixels of the peak-minus-background intensity of the selected Auger peak. The SAM images collected by using the peak-minus-background of the Cr $L_3M_{23}M_{45}$ and N KLL peaks are shown in Figure 12. The black points indicate the area without signal, whereas the lighter grayscale points indicate the area where the signals were detected. As it can be noticed, the layers are well-defined, and the interface is rather neat, suggesting the absence of diffusion phenomena during the deposition process. The coating thickness, estimated from the SEM/SAM images, was about 4.0 µm.

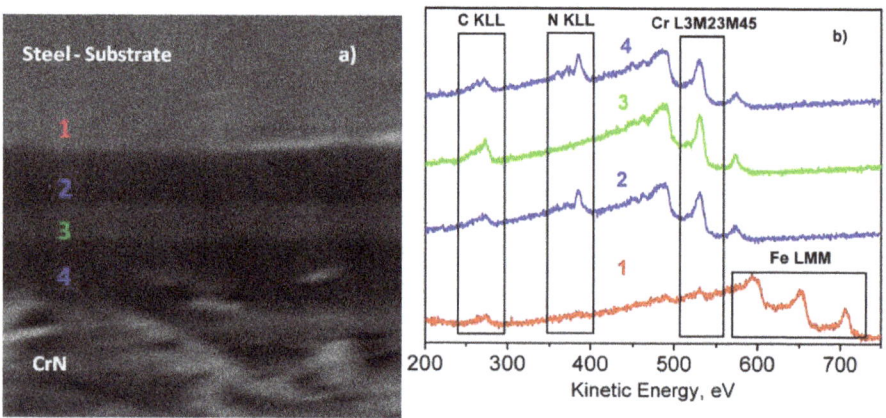

Figure 11. SEM image (**a**) and AES spectra (**b**) acquired along the cross section of the multilayer coating [23].

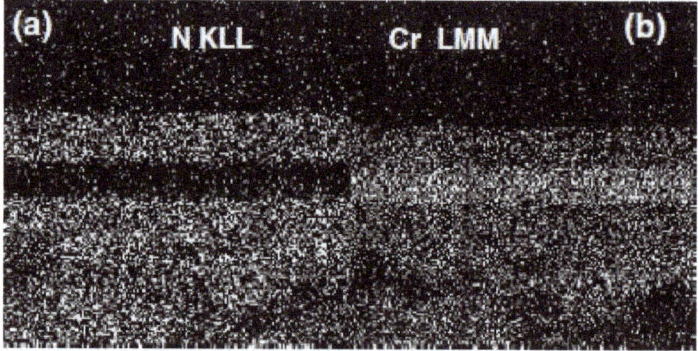

Figure 12. N (**a**) and Cr (**b**) chemical maps of the cross section of multilayer coating [23].

3.3. Microchemical Composition of Ni-Based Superalloys

Superalloys are a class of materials that find numerous applications in the metallurgical field, in particular when a high strength, superior oxidation, and corrosion resistance at temperatures above 700 °C are aquired. Many of superalloys properties are determined by their microstructure, and therefore it is quite important to predict the microstructural evolution during long-time operation, especially the coarsening and morphological changes of the γ' phase that take place at the operating temperature of 800–900 °C. These superalloys are composed of cuboidal γ' particles with submicrometric dimensions, embedded in the γ matrix. The chemical composition of two phases could be different, but most of the previous experimental studies have been dedicated to the morphology and microstructure of superalloys, e.g., [24,25] and the references therein. Practically, the data on the chemical composition of the two phases in various superalloys are absent in the literature. However, the coarsening of γ' particles strongly depends on the difference of chemical composition between a disordered matrix and cuboidal particles. Since this change must occur at the microscale, the surface investigations of the microchemical structure of a biphasic ($\gamma + \gamma'$) Ni-based CM186 superalloy were performed at a high lateral resolution by using the laboratory of scanning photoemission microscopy (SPEM) at the Elettra synchrotron (Trieste, Italy). This technique allows us to directly acquire the surface chemical maps of constituent elements and to determine the variation of their atomic concentrations, eventually induced by the creep tests. In order to prepare for SPEM investigations, the XPS spectra were collected and processed by using a standard XPS apparatus [26,27].

The spectral region, containing all 4f photoemission peaks of constituent elements together with the overlapping peaks of W 5p and Re 5p, is shown in Figure 13.

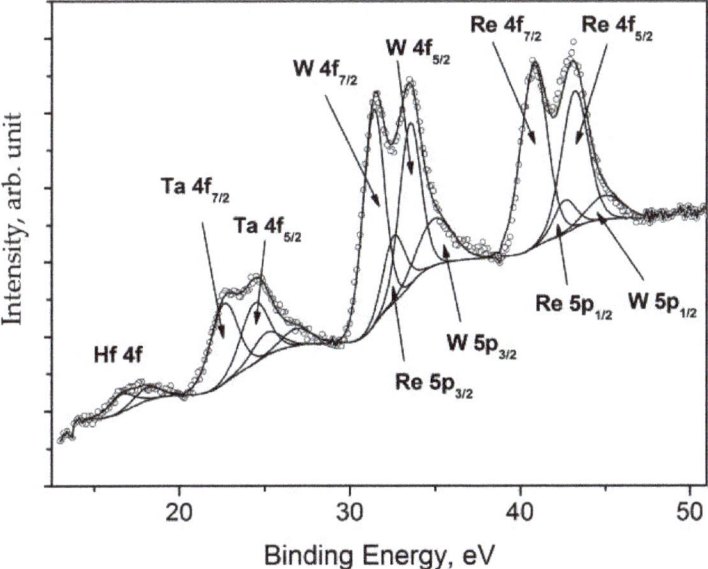

Figure 13. XPS spectrum of the 4f region acquired for the sample of CM186 superalloy [26].

The peak fitting analysis revealed that Re $4f_{7/2}$ and W $4f_{7/2}$ peaks were located at BE = 40.8 and 31.4 eV, corresponding to their metallic states, whereas the Ta $4f_{7/2}$ peak was characterized by two components at 22.6 eV and 25.1 eV, assigned to metallic and oxidized species [26], respectively. Finally, the peak of Hf $4f_{7/2}$ at BE = 16.5 eV was assigned to oxidized species [26].

The chemical maps were recorded in different zones of the samples before and after the creep test, shedding light on the compositional differences between γ and γ' phases. After the acquisition, each map was numerically processed in order to remove the contribution of surface morphology from the photoemission signals. It is worth noting that in SPEM the chemical images can be acquired without any chemical etching of the samples, which is the contrary of the standard microscopies (SEM, AFM, etc.) used for superalloys. Figure 14 shows some examples of obtained chemical maps. The Re 4f, W 4f, and Ta 4f images were acquired from the interdendritic zone on the as-received sample.

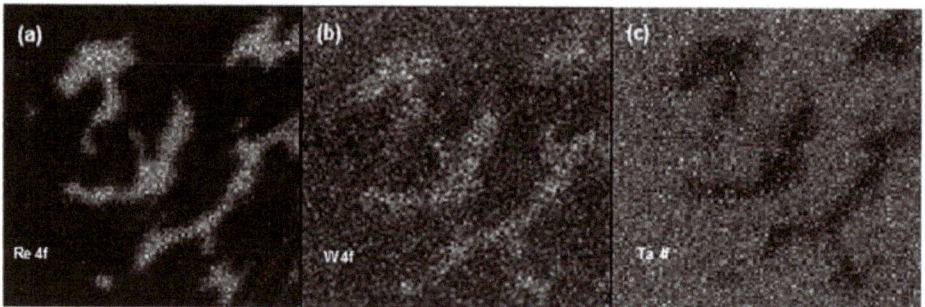

Figure 14. Re 4f (**a**), W 4f (**b**), and Ta 4f (**c**) chemical maps (6.4 × 6.4 µm^2) acquired on the interdendritic zone of the as-received sample [26].

The chemical maps of Re and Ta were complementary, namely, the bright zones in the Re map corresponds to the black zones in that of Ta and vice versa, whereas the tungsten was distributed homogeneously through the analyzed area, even if its content was slightly higher in the γ phase. The lateral distribution of Re and Ta did not change in the crept sample (Figure 15), since they were concentrated in γ and γ' phases, respectively. In comparison with the as-received sample, the distribution of W after creep appeared more uniform. The relative distribution of the main constituent elements between the γ and γ' phases in the as-received and crept samples is displayed in Figure 16. Each data point is the average value of 5 measurements carried out on different points of the same phase. As it can be noticed, both the phases were characterized by the same amount of Ni, while the concentration of Co and Re was predominant in the γ phase.

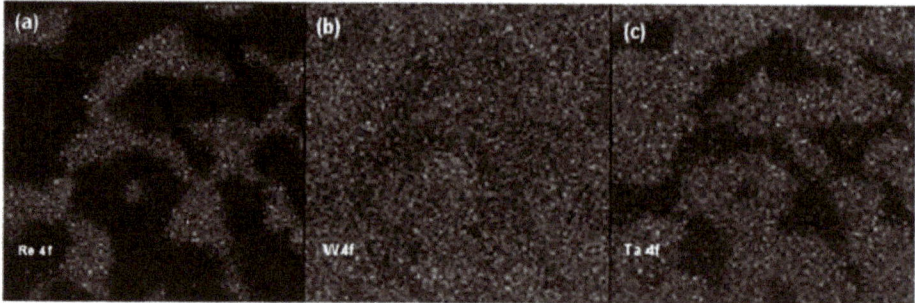

Figure 15. Re 4f (**a**), W 4f (**b**), and Ta 4f (**c**) chemical maps (5.1 × 5.1 µm^2) of the sample after the creep test [26].

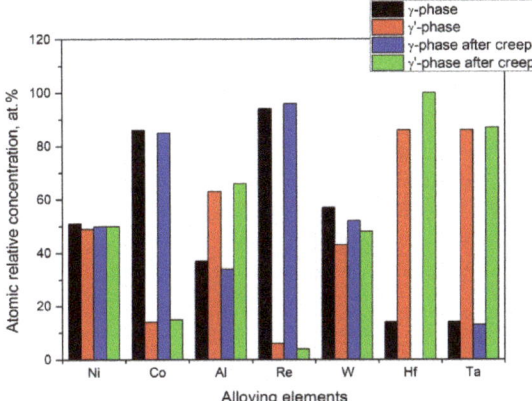

Figure 16. Elemental distribution between the γ and γ' phases before and after the creep test.

After the creep test, their distribution remained almost the same. On the contrary, the amount of Al and Ta was predominant in the γ' phase, remaining unchanged after the creep test. Significant differences were found for W and Hf, where the creep test induced a migration of these elements from the γ phase to γ' phase. The obtained results evidenced that this diffusion process is responsible for the weakening of the disordered matrix during the creep.

3.4. Diffusion Phenomena in the Ti_6Al_4V/SiC_f Composite

There are only a few analytical techniques capable of investigating the diffusion mechanism of the elements in a solid-state sample. Among them, the surface analysis techniques represent the most powerful tool of the investigation, especially in the proximity of the interface between different materials. In this section, we illustrate the multitechnique approach applied for the investigation of a composite material consisting of a Ti_6Al_4V matrix and SiC fibers [28–32].

To avoid the formation of brittle compounds like Ti_5Si_3 at the interface matrix/fiber, each fiber was coated with a 3 µm thick graphite layer. However, at the high temperatures during the fabrication process and in-service life, some elemental diffusion could be induced, reducing the mechanical performance of the composite. Figure 17 shows the elemental distribution on the cross section of the sample.

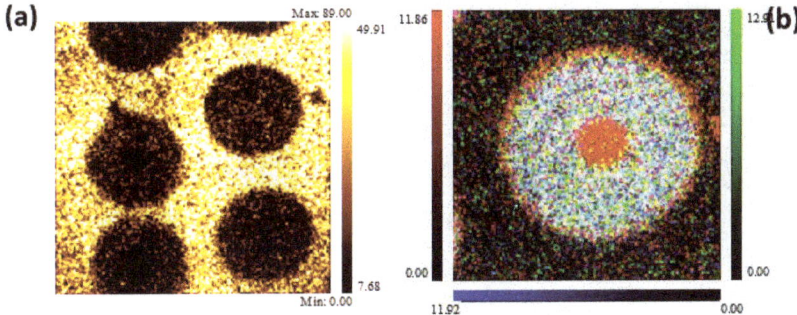

Figure 17. XPS images: (**a**) Ti 2p—400 × 400 µm^2; (**b**) Si 2p (blue), C 1s—190 × 190 µm^2, carbide (green) and graphite (red) [29].

The XPS chemical maps were acquired by collecting the intensity of the signals positioned at BE = 458.8 eV (Ti $2p_{3/2}$), BE = 529.0 eV (O 1s), BE = 99.9 eV (Si 2p), and the intensity of C 1s, where the contributions of graphite (BE = 284.6 eV) and carbide (BE = 283.0 eV) were separated. As it can be seen, the fibers were embedded in the Ti_6Al_4V matrix, which the surface contained oxidized Ti species due to the reaction with atmospheric oxygen. The layer of titanium oxides was promptly removed after a brief time of ion sputtering, reducing the Ti chemical state to metallic one. Unfortunately, the lateral resolution of the standard XPS imaging (>3 µm) was too low for us to investigate the diffusion processes that can occur at the interface matrix/fiber. Therefore, the investigation at a higher lateral resolution was performed by an AES multipoint analysis. SEM images and AES line scan spectra acquired for Samples 1 (as prepared) and 2 (heated for 1000 h at 600 °C) are displayed in Figures 18 and 19, respectively.

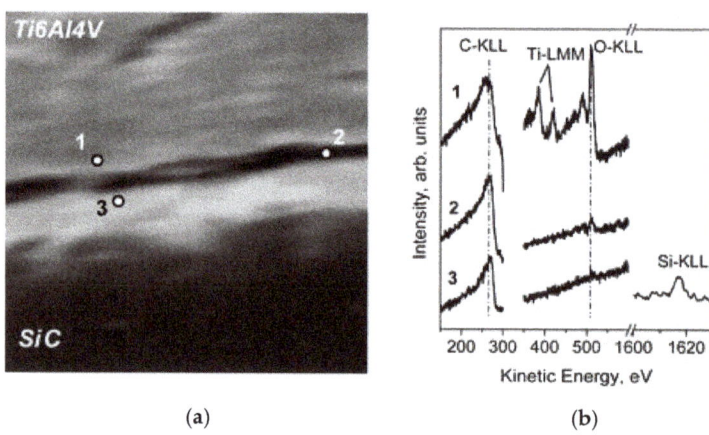

Figure 18. SEM image 80 × 80 µm² (**a**) and AES spectra (**b**) acquired on the cross section of the sample 1 across the carbon layer; analysis points are labelled 1, 2, and 3 [29].

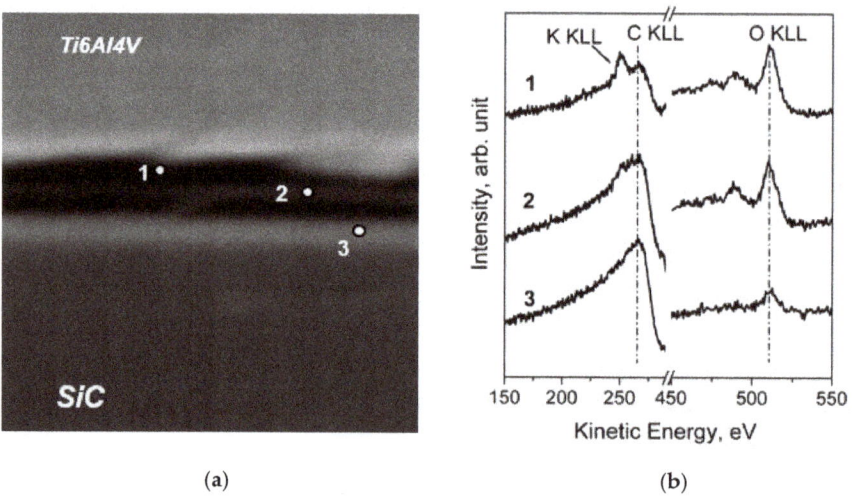

Figure 19. SEM image 80 × 80 µm² (**a**) and AES spectra (**b**) acquired on the cross section of Sample 2 across the carbon layer; analysis points are labelled 1, 2 and 3 [29].

The obtained results revealed that the graphite layer acts as a good protection barrier, avoiding the diffusion of Si in the Ti matrix. However, as evidenced by the SEM analysis, the morphology of the graphite layer became irregular after a thermal treatment at 600 °C for 1000 h, despite its thickness remaining unchanged. This result can be explained by taking into consideration the reaction between carbon and atmospheric oxygen in producing CO. However, the carbon diffusion in the Ti matrix should also be considered. Since the samples have a curvy geometry, the resolution of standard XPS and AES was not sufficient to characterize the chemical species at the interface. To solve this problem, the interface between the graphite and the metallic alloy was investigated by covering the Ti$_6$Al$_4$V and Ti 99.99+ foils with a thin layer of graphite. In order to simulate the diffusion of carbon, the samples were heated in vacuum for 8 h at 500 °C (Figure 20). The XPS depth profiles demonstrated the diffusion of elemental carbon in the metallic matrix, forming a thin layer (about 10 nm) of carbides (Figure 21).

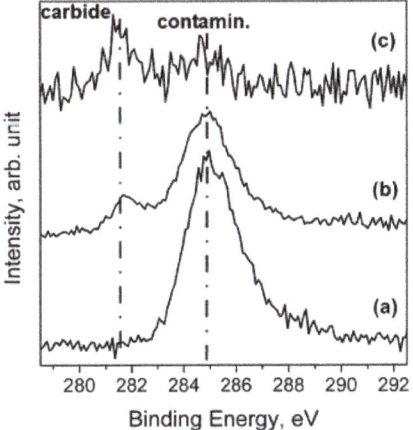

Figure 20. Comparison of C 1s spectra of the (**a**) as-prepared Ti 99.99+ sample; (**b**) Ti 99.99+ sample after 30 min of thermal process at 500 °C; (**c**) Ti 99.99+ sample after 140 min of ion sputtering at 1 keV [29].

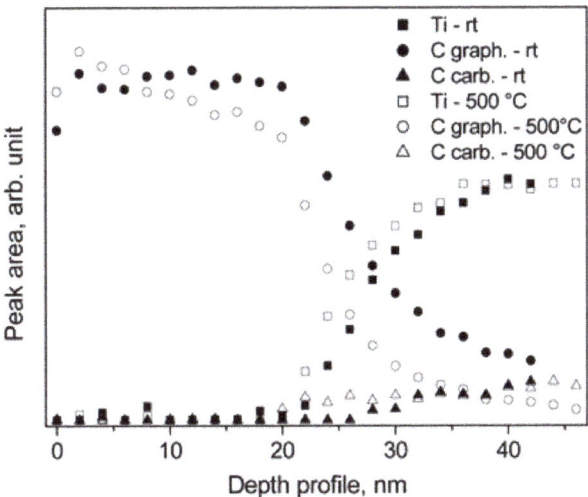

Figure 21. XPS depth profiles of the Ti 99.99+ sample covered with carbon at room temperature (rt) and after heating at 500 °C [29].

From the SPEM analyses [32], carried out on the composite samples, it was concluded that the formation of carbides included not only TiC, but also the interstitial–substitutional (i-s) pairs of C–Al and C–V, present in the α phase of the matrix near the fibers.

3.5. Microchemical Structure of the PbBi Liquid Alloy

The development of a new generation of nuclear reactors has involved many aspects of material science. One of them was the investigation of the microchemical inhomogeneities occurring at high temperature in a liquid Pb-Bi eutectic (LBE) alloy. LBE finds its application in the nuclear reactor as a coolant and spallation source of MYRRHA, an accelerator-driven system. Therefore, it is quite important to investigate any changes of the microchemical structure of LBE that may induce corrosion and embrittlement phenomena in the structural materials. The microstructure of the LBE alloy was evaluated using high-temperature X-ray diffraction (HT-XRD) [33], whereas the microchemical composition was investigated by SPEM [34–36].

In this section, we focus our attention on the surface analysis. Generally, by SPEM, only the solid samples can be analyzed; thus, in order to simulate the clustering formation, we used a rapid cooling (quenching) of liquid alloy starting from different temperatures and assumed that the microchemical composition of the liquid was preserved on the surface of the obtained solid LBE alloy. The selected temperatures for quenching were 126 °C (eutectic temperature) and 200, 300, 400, 518, and 700 °C. The surface chemical maps were acquired by measuring the intensity of the Pb $4f_{7/2}$ and Bi $4f_{7/2}$ peaks, positioned at BE = 137.0 and 156.0 eV, respectively.

Before collecting the maps, the carbon and oxygen contaminations were removed, operating a short cycle of Ar+ ion sputtering. Although the Pb and Bi native oxides were not completely removed, they were neglected because they are meaningless for this discussion. For convenience, the chemical maps were displayed, indicating the Pb/Bi atomic ratio (AR), which is more representative to the elemental distribution. Taking a reference value of the nominal atomic ratio of the eutectic alloy Pb/Bi = 0.8, three pixel colors were used to evidence the three different cases: (i) blue—lack of Pb with AR < 0.6, (ii) red—excess of Pb with AR > 1.0, and (iii) yellow—near a nominal ratio of 0.6 < AR < 1.0. After the acquisition, each image was processed by applying the following procedure of the Igor software: (1) elimination of morphology effects from Pb and Bi maps by using the correction (peak minus background)/background and (2) the superposition of obtained maps and conversion to the maps of atomic ratio AR. Obtained maps of the AR (100 × 100 µm² or 50 × 50 µm²) processed by MATLAB software are presented in Figure 22. As it can be noted, a strong inhomogeneity was observed. Depending on the quenching temperature, Pb and Bi atoms formed the clusters of different dimensions enriched in Bi and/or Pb. At an eutectic temperature, the surface of the sample was characterized by the presence of micrometer clusters enriched in Bi (~90% of Bi), immersed in the alloy with eutectic composition. Increasing the quenching temperature, the elemental distribution and atomic concentration in the clusters were changed. The clusters size was reduced to a few microns (1–5 µm) as the consequence of higher thermal agitation and these clusters were alternatively enriched in Pb and Bi, and the surface distribution of the alloy with an eutectic composition 0.6 < AR < 1.0 was also changed. The cross-section mapping of the sample that was quenched at 518 °C (see Figure 22f) demonstrates how the cooling process was freezing the sample surface in a structure quite similar to the liquid alloy, while the interior of the sample experienced a different temperature gradient, giving rise to the big clusters enriched in Bi. In order to quantify and compare the elemental distribution in different samples, a statistical calculation of the cumulative area CA was applied:

$$CA(AR_i) = \frac{100}{n} \sum_n p_i(AR_i), \qquad (3)$$

where n is the total number of selected pixels p_i that have AR_i in the chemical map.

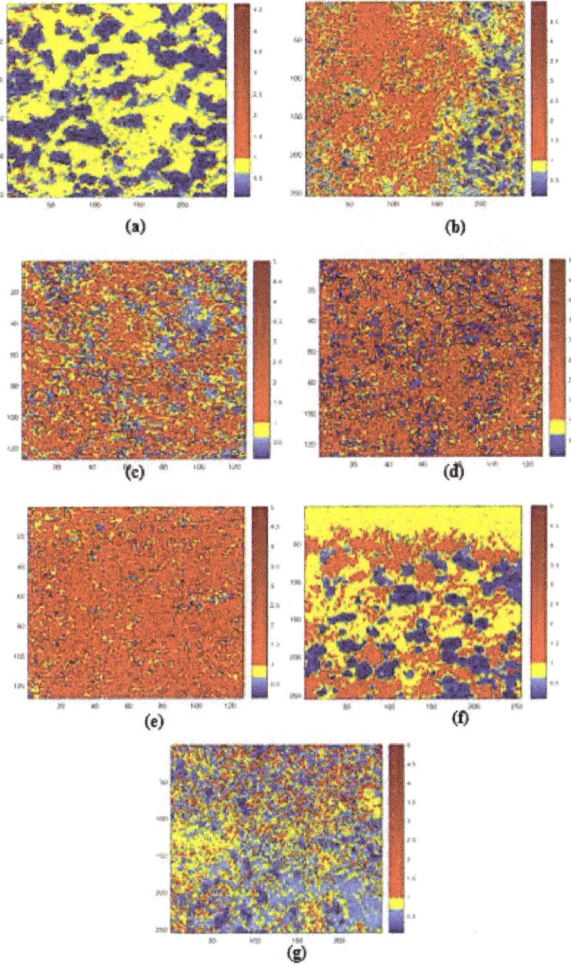

Figure 22. Scanning photoelectron microscopy (SPEM) images of the Pb/Bi atomic ratio (AR) distribution for the samples quenched at (**a**) 126 °C, (**b**) 200 °C, (**c**) 313 °C, (**d**) 401 °C, (**e**) 518 °C, (**f**) 518 °C (cross section of the sample), (**g**) 700 °C.

Figure 23 shows the plot of cumulative area (CA) versus the quenching temperature (QT), where the curves were calculated for AR1, AR2, and AR3. At the melting temperature (126 °C), the CA value of AR2 was approximately 2.5%, indicating a very low concentration of Pb, whereas the CA values of AR1 and AR3 were almost similar at 52% and 45%, respectively. Increasing QT, the CA of AR2 was augmenting almost linearly until over 80% at QT = 600 °C, then suddenly falling down below 10% at QT = 700 °C. The comparison of these curves with the phase transition determined by HT-XRD investigations confirmed that the structural modification is also accompanied by the change of the number of clusters enriched in Pb (AR2). As regards the curves of AR1 and AR3, they substantially showed a complementary trend with respect to the AR2 one.

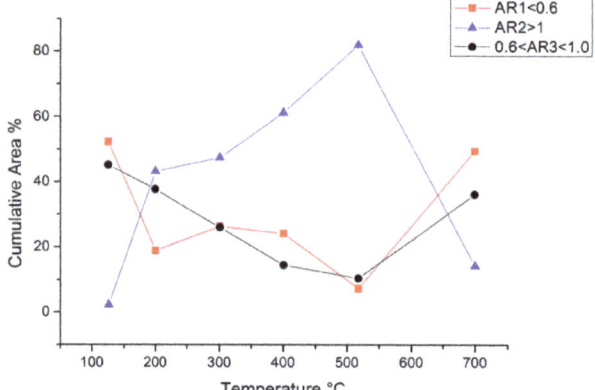

Figure 23. Cumulative area (CA) vs. quenching temperature for the three ranges of atomic ratio (AR): the values of AR1, AR2, and AR3.

3.6. Austenitic Steels

Austenitic stainless steels are known as materials with a high corrosion resistance in different environments. Because of their low hardness, however, they cannot be used in several industrial applications, unless after modifications through thermochemical surface treatments. Carburizing, nitriding, and carbo-nitriding are common examples of the heat treatments that are used to increase the hardness of stainless steels. These processes need to reach a temperature higher than 550 °C, which could cause the local microstructural changes in the austenitic steel phase, such as the precipitation of Cr carbides. Since these precipitates can reduce the corrosion resistance of the steel, it is necessary to adopt some heat treatment at a lower temperature. A good alternative is the kolstering process, which can harden the austenitic steels without compromising their resistance to corrosion. Although kolstering is a good low-temperature treatment, it is unfortunately very long lasting and expensive. It involves a pretreatment of the steel in an HCl atmosphere at about 250 °C to remove the Cr_2O_3 layer from the surface. Then, the stainless steel is treated at 450 °C in a gaseous atmosphere of CO, H_2, and N_2 for a duration about 30 h.

Very promising results close to those of kolstering were obtained through a plasma carburizing process at low temperature. In the study presented in [37], the plasma was generated by microwaves operating up to 200 mbar as described in detail in [38], while the temperature and pressure were set to about 420 °C and 80 mbar, respectively, for the whole treatment duration of about 6 h. The chamber gas mixture was formed by CH_4 (variable percentage) in H_2. The main advantage of this treatment is the reduction of the process time, and consequently this is more convenient also for process costs.

XPS and AES techniques allow for the study of the steel surface before and after these treatments. In particular, these techniques permit us to examine the chemical composition of the superficial hardened layer. In this way, it is possible to identify the best process condition, for example, by changing some parameters of the treatment. In this study, the percentage of CH_4, added to H_2 in the gas mixture was varied from 2% to 10%.

The results of microhardness tests and XRD measurements [1] have established that the sample treated with 2% of CH_4 was the one with the best results in terms of hardness (700 HV) and corrosion resistance, without the presence of any precipitates of Cr carbides. For a better understanding of these results, all the samples were investigated by surface analysis.

An AES line scan over the cross section, shown in Figure 24a, revealed the presence of an additional carbon layer with a thickness of about 2–3 µm (lighter zone) above the hardened layer of 20 µm. As it is possible to see from Figure 24b, the Auger signals of C KLL, O KLL, Cr LMM, and Fe LMM were detected along the whole cross section. In the first point, corresponding to the zone near the surface, the amount of carbon is the highest, and the concentrations of Fe and Cr are low. The ratio of the signals intensity (Fe LMM)/(C KLL) is equal to 0.5. Instead, at the point closest to the bulk, the amount of carbon returns to the nominal value of the alloy, and the ratio Fe/C is equal to 0.9. The intensity ratio of (Fe LMM)/(C KLL) for the entire line scan is shown in Figure 25.

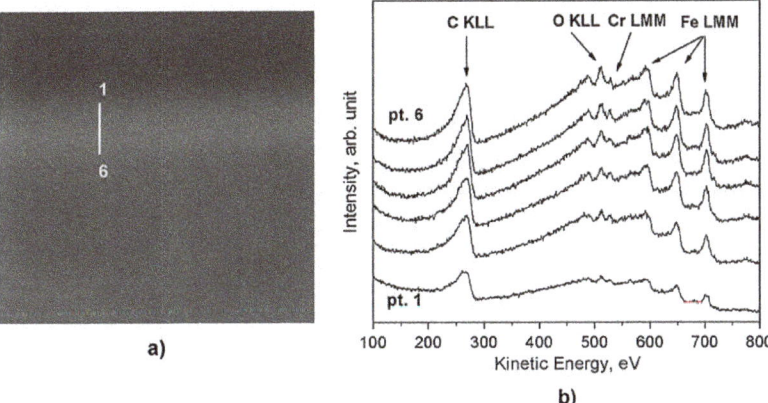

Figure 24. SEM image (24 × 24 μm^2) of the sample treated by plasma at CH$_4$ 2% in H$_2$ (**a**), and Auger spectra (**b**) recorded in points 1–6 are marked in the SEM image [37].

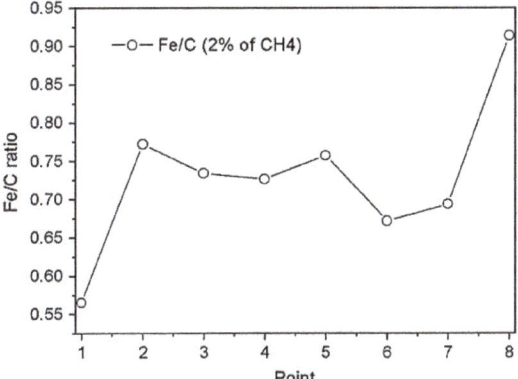

Figure 25. (Fe LMM)/(C KLL) intensity ratio calculated along the line scan. [37].

From the value of the D parameter, which is the distance between the most positive maximum and the most negative minimum of the first derivative of C KLL spectrum [39], it is possible to establish that the samples subjected to carburization with a gas mixture composed of 2% of CH$_4$ and H$_2$ have a ultrathin outer layer of graphitic nature (C–C bond with a majority of planar sp^2 hybridization). Because of the presence of this additional hard graphitic layer, which was not present in the other samples treated with higher percentages of CH$_4$, it is possible to conclude that 2% of CH$_4$ is the best gas mixture process condition. In this way, the hardened surface of the austenitic steel is comparable to the one obtained with the kolstering treatment.

Another interesting discovery of austenitic steels that has been reported in the papers [40,41], concerns the microstructural modification in the steel with a high content of N (about 0.8 wt.%) induced by heating. Although nitrogen stabilizes the austenitic phase and increases the corrosion resistance, it is important to note that N is soluble only for quantities less than 0.4 wt.% (both in the liquid and solid phase). After exceeding this value, the discontinuous precipitations of chromium nitride are formed in the steel in the range of temperature between 700 and 900 °C.

The transformation that occurs during heat treatments in that temperature range is the following:

$$\gamma_s \rightarrow \gamma + Cr_2N, \tag{4}$$

where γ_s is the N-supersaturated austenitic phase (initial phase of the steel), γ is the austenitic transformed phase which appears as a lamellar structure, and Cr_2N is the chromium nitride precipitates. A SEM image with the corresponding schematic structure of the austenitic steel is shown in Figure 26.

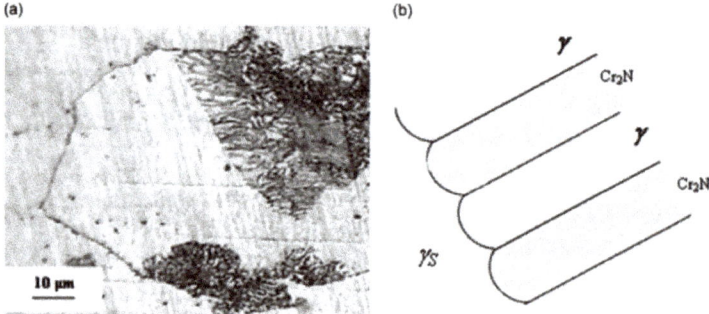

Figure 26. SEM image of partially transformed austenitic grain after 2 h at 850 °C (**a**) and a schematic of the structure (**b**) [40].

As it is explained in much detail in the cited papers [40,41], there were some experimental evidences, such as XRD reflection peaks as well as the values of the microhardness and lattice parameter in the transformed and untransformed zones, which suggested the presence of a net flow of nitrogen from the untransformed N-supersaturated γ_s zones to γ, along the precipitation process. Therefore, XPS and AES techniques could be used to establish final evidence of this phenomenon.

As it is possible to see from Figure 26a, the grains size of γ_s is about 100 μm, while the dimension of the transformed areas is much smaller, at about 10 μm. A traditional XPS apparatus is not adequate for us to study the chemical composition of the transformed zones with sufficient resolution because it can analyze only surface areas between 0.1 and 1 mm. For this reason, it was necessary to use a scanning photoelectron microscopy (SPEM) operating in both imaging and spectroscopy modes. Indeed, this type of analysis can use an X-ray microprobe with a diameter less than 100 nm.

By using the SPEM technique, it was possible to determine the chemical composition and spatial distribution of the elements in the lamellae and interlamellar spaces. In Figure 27, a spatially resolved XPS image of the transformed zone before and after the topographical correction is shown.

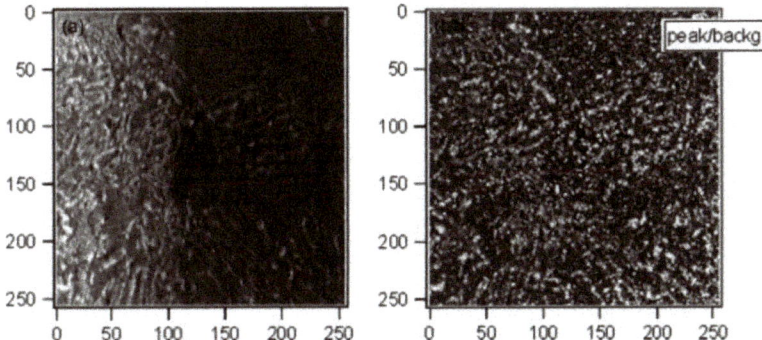

Figure 27. SPEM Cr 3p chemical images (51.2 × 51.2 μm^2) of the sample treated for 23 h at 850 °C: (**a**) as-acquired and (**b**) corrected for the sample topography by calculating the ratio peak/background for Cr 3p signal [40].

The information obtained from these images and from the microscopy was in good agreement with traditional XPS measurements. From the SPEM images of Cr 3p signal, it was found that in the transformed zone, Cr is concentrated in the lamellae, whereas it is uniformly distributed in low concentration in the untransformed region. In an opposite way to Cr distribution, a Fe-enrichment in the untransformed zone and impoverishment in the lamellae were revealed from Fe 3p images. These analyses indicate a migration of Cr, which is mainly accumulated in the Cr$_2$N precipitates across the interface between γ and γ_s.

Furthermore, from the Auger spectra shown in Figure 28, the Cr/N atomic ratio was calculated. It was found to be equal to 2.9 and 5.9 for the transformed and untransformed zones, respectively. This result confirms the nitrogen enrichment in the transformed zones during the heat treatment. Moreover, another phenomenon was also explained. In fact, from these analyses it was possible to hypothesize that the precipitation of Cr$_2$N takes place as long as the flow of nitrogen from the untransformed to the transformed area is present. Finally, when γ and γ_s zones have the same concentration of N, the precipitation process is stopped, even if not all the cells of the steel were transformed.

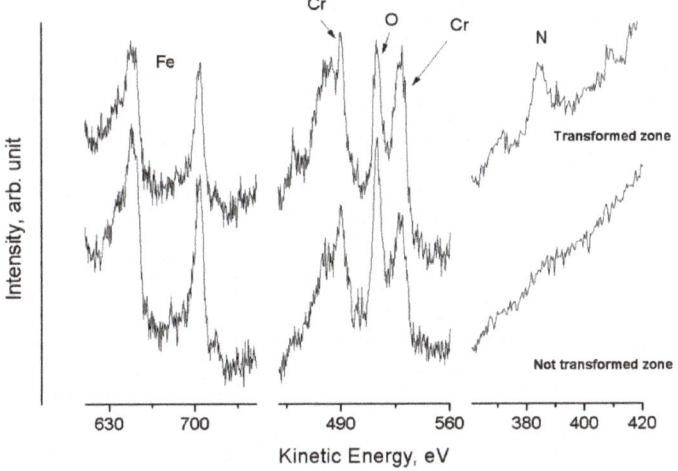

Figure 28. Auger spectra (Fe LMM, Cr LMM, O KLL, and N KLL) of untransformed and transformed zones of the steel sample after 23 h at 850 °C [40].

3.7. Graphene on Polycrystalline Metals

The last few decades of material science will be remembered as the years of the graphene revolution. In fact, although the theoretical predictions can be traced starting from the 19th century, the experimental evidences occurred only in the 2004. After that, throughout the scientific community there was a continuous race to discover the new fields of application in order to exploit the full potential of this 2D material. At the same time, it was essential to develop an industrial method of synthesis that could guarantee a large-scale production of graphene.

Recently, the research for the development of microelectronic devices, transparent conductive films, and in general different type of sensors with graphene has focused on the growth of graphene via the chemical vapor deposition (CVD) on polycrystalline metal substrates. These substrates act as excellent catalysts for the epitaxial growth of graphene. Some of them are also cheap and are easily removable, when it is necessary to transfer the layer of graphene on the device where it has to operate [42,43].

Numerous studies, extensively reviewed in [42–45], have been dedicated to the growth and characterization of graphene on various metals. Among many analytical techniques for the characterization of graphene, the mostly attractive ones are Raman spectroscopy, atomic force, and transmission electron microscopies, XPS and AES. However, in many papers including those on XPS, only the photoemission spectrum of C 1s has been used for graphene characterization, even if it does not allow the main peaks of graphene and graphite to be differentiated [44,46] without the angle-resolved analysis of low intensity σ and π bands accompanying the main peak [45]. A more useful and easier approach is the unequivocal identification of graphene from the analysis of C KVV spectrum combined with the main photoemission peaks of substrate and C 1s [46]. This approach, combined with Raman spectroscopy, allows us to obtain the information on the uniformity of graphene layer over a large area. In the same manner, these analyses permit us to determine the graphene thickness, which can often differ from the monolayer. The parameters, as well as the morphology and the thickness, depend on the type of growth mechanism of graphene. In the case of the CVD technique, two different growth mechanisms can take place: the decomposition of hydrocarbon gas at high temperature or the segregation of C atoms on the metal surface during the cooling phase.

For example, in the study in [47], the graphene was synthesized on the substrates of various polycrystalline metals. The growth was carried out by the CVD technique in a mixture of CH_4-H_2 gas at 1000 °C, with different times of exposure to the gas: 2, 4, and 6 min for the Cu substrate; and only 2 min for the Ni-Cu alloy (20 wt.% of Cu) and pure Ni film on Si substrate.

It was possible to make a preliminary test of graphene quality by Raman spectroscopy. At first, the disorder degree of the deposited films can be estimated from the intensity of the D-band (1350 cm^{-1}). Then, the ratio of the G-peaks band (1582 cm^{-1}) was calculated due to the presence of graphite or a multilayer system of graphene with respect to the typical signal of graphene G′-band (2700 cm^{-1}). The Raman spectra of graphene deposited on Cu foils are shown in Figure 29.

As it was observed from the value of the IG′/IG ratio, the sample exposed for 6 min to the gas mixture at 1000 °C appeared to be the most promising. This result was also confirmed by photoemission measurements.

Because it is not possible to distinguish between the graphite and graphene (both peaks are positioned at BE of about 284.5 eV) from the C 1s photoemission spectra, the Auger spectra of C KLL were also acquired. In fact, from the calculation of the D parameter, i.e., the distance between the absolute maximum and the absolute minimum of the first derivative of C KLL spectrum [39], it is possible to identify the presence of graphene [46]. Therefore, the value of D parameter was determined from the C KLL spectra induced by an X-ray source (XAES) and then it was compared with the same parameter obtained by using excitation with an electron gun (AES).

The typical spectra of C 1s and C KLL regions are shown in Figure 30, whereas all the results of the XPS characterization are summarized in the Tables 2–4.

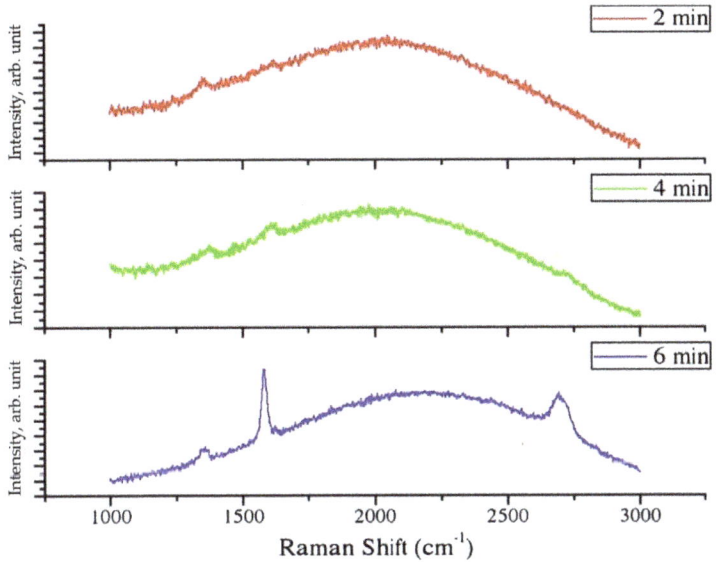

Figure 29. Raman spectra of graphene grown on electroformed Cu foils: exposure time of 2, 4, and 6 min [47].

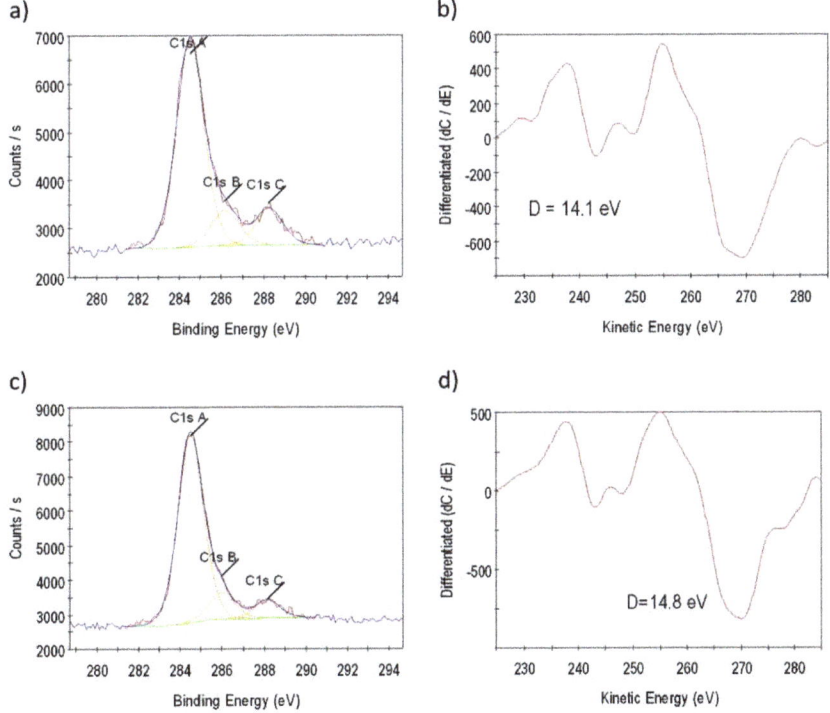

Figure 30. XPS spectra of C 1s for the samples 4 (**a**) and 6 (**c**) grown on Cu at 1000 °C. The corresponding C KLL spectra in the first derivative are shown in (**b**) and (**d**), respectively [47].

Table 2. Summary of XPS results for Sample 4 of graphene on Cu substrate [47].

Sample 4 Peak	BE, eV	FWHM, eV	Atomic %	Bond
C1s A	284.5	1.51	44.1	C–C (graphene or graphite)
C1s B	286.2	1.51	7.4	C–O
C1s C	288.3	1.51	7.7	Carboxyl O–C=O
Cu2$p_{3/2}$ A	932.5	1.71	9.3	Cu(0)
Cu2$p_{3/2}$ B	934.7	1.71	1.6	Cu(OH)$_2$
O1s A	530.7	1.87	6.1	C–O
O1s B	531.8	1.87	20.9	OH groups, C=O
Cl2p	199.0	1.41	2.8	-

Table 3. Summary of XPS results for Sample 6 of graphene on Cu substrate [47].

Sample 6 Peak	BE, eV	FWHM, eV	Atomic %	Bond
C1s A	284.5	1.42	51.8	C–C (graphene or graphite)
C1s B	286.0	1.42	7.2	C–O
C1s C	288.2	1.42	5.2	Carboxyl O–C=O
Cu2$p_{3/2}$ A	932.4	1.51	12.8	Cu(0)
Cu2$p_{3/2}$ B	934.6	1.51	1.2	Cu(OH)$_2$
O1s A	530.5	1.61	8.3	C–O
O1s B	531.8	1.61	12.3	OH groups, C=O
Cl2p	199.0	1.50	1.2	-

Table 4. D parameter (eV) determined by XPS and XAES for graphene samples on Cu substrate [47].

Experimental	Sample 4	Sample 6	Description
XPS at 90°	14.1	1.42	Diamond-like
XPS at 45°	13.3	14.2	Diamond-like
XAES (e$^-$ beam)	22.1	21.5	Graphitic

From the Table 3, it is possible to conclude that the best graphene sample was obtained by the deposition of 6 min: The obtained values of the D parameter were D_{XAES} = 14.1 eV (diamond-like) and D_{AES} = 22.1 eV (graphitic) (see Table 4). As it was explained in detail in the previous work [46], these values definitely indicate the presence of graphene. From the XPS measurements at the grazing angle, it was also estimated that the thickness of graphene film was equal to a few monolayers.

In this way, a further example of the application of surface spectroscopic techniques demonstrated their versatility and potentiality in recent fields of scientific research and industrial development, such as the large-scale production of graphene.

4. Summary

The importance and potentiality of ESCA techniques for the exploration of metallic surfaces was illustrated by reviewing the main principles of these techniques and seven experimental cases of our research. The main techniques comprised in ESCA, i.e., X-ray photoemission and Auger electron spectroscopies, were successfully employed for the investigation of different metallic surfaces, and their modifications were induced by different treatments or operating conditions. In addition, the high resolution SPEM technique was applied for the exploration of submicrometric features of surface chemical composition in some of investigated materials.

Various phenomena on the metallic surfaces were revealed: the formation of impurity defects on collection coins, the microchemical composition and corrosion of stainless steel coated by Cr and Ti nitrides, modifications of microchemical composition in biphasic Ni-based superalloys, carbon diffusion at high temperature in the interface of Ti6Al4V/SiCf composite, microchemical inhomogeneity of liquid PbBi alloy, surface modification of austenitic steels by plasma carburizing, and nitrogen migration at high temperature, with an influence of polycrystalline metal substrates (Cu, Ni, and NiCu alloy) on the growth of graphene. One more recent example of an advantageous ESCA application for the study of Cr segregation in martensitic stainless steel is reported in the present issue of this journal [48].

Author Contributions: Conceptualization, E.B., S.K., and A.M.; investigation, E.B., S.K., and A.M.; writing and editing, E.B., S.K., and A.M.; All authors have read and agreed to the published version of the manuscript.

Funding: No funding has been received for preparation of this review.

Acknowledgments: The authors are grateful to all the coauthors of reviewed papers for their contributions. Our special thanks are dedicated to Roberto Montanari (Tor Vergata University of Rome), who initiated the research in a major part of the reviewed cases, also to Luca Gregoratti and his team for hosting us at the ESCA microscopy beamline in the Elettra synchrotron and providing extensive experimental support.

Conflicts of Interest: The authors declare no conflict of interest.

References

1. Hagström, S.; Nordling, C.; Siegbahn, K. Electron spectroscopy for chemical analyses. *Phys. Lett.* **1964**, *9*, 235–236. [CrossRef]
2. Fahlman, A.; Hamrin, K.; Nordberg, R.; Nordling, C.; Siegbahn, K. Revision of Electron Binding Energies in Light Elements. *Phys. Rev. Lett.* **1965**, *14*, 127–129. [CrossRef]
3. Carlson, T.A.; Mcguire, G.E. Study of the x-ray photoelectron spectrum of tungsten—Tungsten oxide as a function of thickness of the surface oxide layer. *J. Electron Spectrosc. Relal. Phenom.* **1972**, *1*, 161–168. [CrossRef]
4. Schön, G.; Lundin, S.T. ESCA studies of oxygen adsorption on nickel. *J. Electron Spectrosc. Rel.Phenom.* **1972**, *1*, 105–109. [CrossRef]
5. Moulder, J.F.; Stickle, W.F.; Sobol, P.E.; Bomben, K.D. *Handbook of X-ray Photoelectron Spectroscopy*; Phys. Electronics Inc.: Eden Prairie, MN, USA, 1992.
6. Childs, K.D.; Carlson, B.A.; LaVanier, L.A.; Moulder, J.F.; Paul, D.F.; Stickle, W.F.; Watson, D.G. *Handbook of Auger Electron Spectroscopy*; Phys. Electronics Inc.: Eden Prairie, MN, USA, 1995.
7. Feuerbacher, B.; Fitton, B.; Willis, R.F. *Photoemission and the Electronic Properties of Surfaces*; J. Wiley & Sons: Chichester, UK, 1978.
8. Briggs, D.; Seah, M.P. *Practical Surface Analysis Auger and X-ray Photoelectron Spectroscopy*, 2nd ed.; J. Wiley & Sons: Chichester, UK, 1990.
9. De Crescenzi, M.; Piancastelli, M.N. *Electron Scattering and Rel. Spectroscopies*; World Scientific Publishing: Singapore, 1996.
10. Lindgren, I. Chemical shifts in X-ray and photo-electron spectroscopy: A historical review. *J. Electron Spectrosc. Rel. Phenom.* **2004**, *137*, 59–71. [CrossRef]
11. X-ray Photoelectron Spectroscopy. Available online: https://mmrc.caltech.edu/SS_XPS/XPS_PPT/XPS_Slides.pdf (accessed on 17 November 2020).
12. Walton, J. Quantitative surface chemical microscopy by X-ray photoelectron spectroscopy. *Spectrosc. Eur.* **2007**, *19/6*, 7–10.
13. McIntyre, N.S.; Davidson, R.D.; Kim, G.; Francis, J.T. New frontiers in X-ray photoelectron spectroscopy. *Vacuum* **2003**, *69*, 63–71. [CrossRef]
14. Gunther, S.; Kaulich, B.; Gregoratti, L.; Kiskinova, M. Photoelectron microscopy and applications in surface and materials science. *Prog. Surf. Sci.* **2002**, *70*, 187–260. [CrossRef]
15. Potts, A.W.; Morrison, G.R.; Gregoratti, L.; Barinov, A.; Kaulich, B.; Kiskinova, M. The exploitation of multichannel detection in scanning photoemission microscopy. *Surf. Rev. Lett.* **2002**, *9*, 705–708. [CrossRef]
16. Gusmano, G.; Montanari, R.; Kaciulis, S.; Montesperelli, G.; Denk, R. Gold corrosion: Red stains on a gold Austrian Ducat. *Appl. Phys. A* **2004**, *79*, 205–211. [CrossRef]
17. Gusmano, G.; Montanari, R.; Kaciulis, S.; Mezzi, A.; Montesperelli, G.; Rupprecht, L. Surface defects on collection coins of precious metals. *Surf. Interface Anal.* **2004**, *36*, 921–924. [CrossRef]

18. Moretti, G. Auger parameter and Wagner plot in the characterization of chemical states by X-ray photoelectron spectroscopy: A review. *J. Electron Spectrosc. Rel. Phenom.* **1998**, *95*, 95–144. [CrossRef]
19. Ingo, G.M.; Kaciulis, S.; Mezzi, A.; Valente, T.; Gusmano, G. Surface characterization of titanium nitride composite coatings fabricated by reactive plasma spraying. *Surf. Interface Anal.* **2004**, *36*, 1147–1150. [CrossRef]
20. Ingo, G.M.; Kaciulis, S.; Mezzi, A.; Valente, T.; Casadei, F.; Gusmano, G. Characterization of composite titanium nitride coatings prepared by reactive plasma spraying. *Electrochim. Acta.* **2005**, *50*, 4531–4537. [CrossRef]
21. Caballero, A.; Leinen, D.; Espinos, J.P.; Fernandez, A.; Gonzalez-Elipe, A.R. Use of XAS and chemical probes to study the structural damage induced in oxide ceramics by bombardment with low-energy ions. *Surf. Interface Anal.* **1994**, *21*, 418–424. [CrossRef]
22. Hashimoto, S.; Hirokawa, K.; Fukuda, Y.; Suzuki, K.; Suzuki, T.; Usuki, N.; Gennai, N.; Yoshida, S.; Koda, M.; Sezaki, H.; et al. Correction of peak shift and classification of change of X-ray photoelectron spectra of oxides as a result of ion sputtering. *Surf. Interface Anal.* **1992**, *18*, 799–806. [CrossRef]
23. Kaciulis, S.; Mezzi, A.; Montesperelli, G.; Lamastra, F.; Rapone, M.; Casadei, F.; Valente, T.; Gusmano, G. Multi-technique study of corrosion resistant CrN/Cr/CrN and CrN: C coatings. *Surf. Coat. Technol.* **2006**, *201*, 313–319. [CrossRef]
24. Monjati, H.; Jahazi, M.; Bahrami, R.; Yue, S. The influence of heat treatment conditions on characteristics in Udimet®720. *Mat. Sci. Eng. A* **2004**, *373*, 286–293. [CrossRef]
25. Ges, A.M.; Fornaro, O.; Palacio, H.A. Coarsening behaviour of a Ni-base superalloy under different heat treatment conditions. *Mat. Sci. Eng. A* **2007**, *458*, 96–100. [CrossRef]
26. Kaciulis, S.; Mezzi, A.; Amati, M.; Montanari, R.; Angella, G.; Maldini, M. Relation between the microstructure and microchemistry in Ni-based superalloy. *Surf. Interface Anal.* **2012**, *44*, 982–985. [CrossRef]
27. Amati, M.; Gregoratti, L.; Balijepalli, S.K.; Kaciulis, S.; Mezzi, A.; Montanari, R.; Angella, G.; Donnini, R.; Maldini, M.; Ripamonti, D. Microchemical analysis through SPEM for a nickel superalloy after creep test. *Metall. Ital.* **2013**, *105*, 21–26.
28. Donnini, R.; Kaciulis, S.; Mezzi, A.; Montanari, R.; Tata, M.E.; Testani, C. MicrO–Chemical characterization of fibermatrix interface in TI6ALAV-SICF composite. Caratterizzazione microchimica dell'interfaccia fibra-matrice nel composito TI6AL4V-SICf. *Metall. Ital.* **2007**, *99*, 13–18.
29. Donnini, R.; Kaciulis, S.; Mezzi, A.; Montanari, R.; Testani, C. Composite of Ti6Al4V and SiC fibres: Evolution of fibre-matrix interface during heat treatments. *Surf. Interface Anal.* **2008**, *40*, 277–280. [CrossRef]
30. Deodati, P.; Donnini, R.; Kaciulis, S.; Mezzi, A.; Montanari, R.; Testani, C.; Ucciardello, N. Anelastic phenomena at the fibre-matrix interface of the Ti6Al4V-SiC f composite. *Key Eng. Mater.* **2010**, *425*, 263–270. [CrossRef]
31. Deodati, P.; Donnini, R.; Kaciulis, S.; Mezzi, A.; Montanari, R.; Testani, C.; Ucciardello, N. Microstructural characterization of Ti6Al4V-SiCf composite produced by new roll-bonding process. *Adv. Mat. Res.* **2010**, *89*, 715–720.
32. Kaciulis, S.; Mezzi, A.; Donnini, R.; Deodati, P.; Montanari, R.; Ucciardello, N.; Amati, M.; KazemianAbyaneh, M.; Testani, C. Microchemical characterisation of carbon-metal interface in Ti6Al4V-SiCf composites. *Surf. Interface Anal.* **2010**, *42*, 707–711. [CrossRef]
33. Montanari, R.; Varone, A. Physical phenomena leading to melting of metals. *Mater. Sci. Forum.* **2017**, *884*, 3–17. [CrossRef]
34. Mezzi, A.; Kaciulis, S.; Balijepalli, S.K.; Montanari, R.; Varone, A.; Amati, M.; Aleman, B. Microchemical inhomogeneity in eutectic Pb-Bi alloy quenched from melt. *Surf. Interface Anal.* **2014**, *46*, 877–881. [CrossRef]
35. Amati, M.; Balijepalli, S.K.; Mezzi, A.; Kaciulis, S.; Montanari, R.; Varone, A. Temperature dependent phenomena in liquid LBE alloy. *Mater. Sci. Forum.* **2017**, *884*, 41–52. [CrossRef]
36. Montanari, R.; Varone, A.; Gregoratti, L.; Kaciulis, S.; Mezzi, A. Lead-bismuth eutectic: Atomic and micro-scale melt evolution. *Materials* **2019**, *12*, 3158. [CrossRef]
37. Ciancaglioni, I.; Donnini, R.; Kaciulis, S.; Mezzi, A.; Montanari, R.; Ucciardello, N.; Verona-Rinati, G. Surface modification of austenitic steels by low-temperature carburization. *Surf. Interface Anal.* **2012**, *44*, 1001–1004. [CrossRef]

38. Bagalà, P.; Gusmano, G.; Montesperelli, G.; Montanari, R.; Ucciardello, N.; Verona-Rinati, G. Valutazione della resistenza alla corrosione di acciai inossidabili ad alto tenore di azoto sensibilizzati ad alta temperature. In *Giornate Nazionali sulla Corrosione e Protezione*; Monte Porzio Catone: Rome, Italy, 2011.
39. Kaciulis, S.; Mezzi, A. Surface investigation of carbon films: From diamond to graphite. *Surf. Interface Anal.* **2010**, *42*, 1082–1084.
40. Carosi, A.; Amati, M.; Gregoratti, L.; Kaciulis, S.; Mezzi, A.; Montanari, R.; Rovatti, L.; Ucciardello, N. Heating modification of an austenitic steel with high-nitrogen content. *Surf. Interface Anal.* **2010**, *42*, 726–729. [CrossRef]
41. Rovatti, L.; Montanari, R.; Ucciardello, N.; Mezzi, A.; Kaciulis, S.; Carosi, A. Discontinuous precipitation in a high-nitrogen austenitic steel. *Mater. Sci. Forum.* **2010**, *638*, 3597–3602. [CrossRef]
42. Mattevi, C.; Kim, H.; Chhowalla, M. A review of chemical vapour deposition of graphene on copper. *J. Mater. Chem.* **2011**, *21*, 3324–3334. [CrossRef]
43. Wintterlin, J.; Bocquet, M.-L. Graphene on metal surfaces. *Surf. Sci.* **2009**, *603*, 1841–1852. [CrossRef]
44. Batzill, M. The surface science of graphene: Metal interfaces, CVD synthesis, nanoribbons, chemical modifications, and defects. *Surf. Sci. Rep.* **2012**, *67*, 83–115. [CrossRef]
45. Algdal, J.; Balasubramanian, T.; Breitholtz, M.; Kihlgren, T.; Walldén, L. Thin graphite overlayers: Graphene and alkali metal intercalation. *Surf. Sci.* **2007**, *601*, 1167–1175. [CrossRef]
46. Kaciulis, S.; Mezzi, A.; Calvani, P.; Trucchi, D.M. Electron spectroscopy of the main allotropes of carbon. *Surf. Interface Anal.* **2014**, *46*, 966–969. [CrossRef]
47. Nobili, L.; Magnin, L.; Bernasconi, R.; Livolsi, F.; Pedrazzetti, L.; Lucotti, A.; Balijepalli, S.K.; Mezzi, A.; Kaciulis, S.; Montanari, R. Investigation of graphene layers on electrodeposited polycrystalline metals. *Surf. Interface Anal.* **2016**, *48*, 456–460. [CrossRef]
48. Bolli, E.; Fava, A.; Ferro, P.; Kaciulis, S.; Mezzi, A.; Montanari, R.; Varone, A. Cr segregation and impact fracture in a martensitic stainless steel. *Coatings* **2020**, *10*, 843. [CrossRef]

Publisher's Note: MDPI stays neutral with regard to jurisdictional claims in published maps and institutional affiliations.

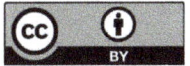

© 2020 by the authors. Licensee MDPI, Basel, Switzerland. This article is an open access article distributed under the terms and conditions of the Creative Commons Attribution (CC BY) license (http://creativecommons.org/licenses/by/4.0/).

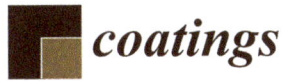

Article

Cr Segregation and Impact Fracture in a Martensitic Stainless Steel

Eleonora Bolli [1,2,*], Alessandra Fava [3], Paolo Ferro [4], Saulius Kaciulis [2], Alessio Mezzi [2], Roberto Montanari [1] and Alessandra Varone [1,*]

1. Department of Industrial Engineering, University of Rome "Tor Vergata", Via del Politecnico 1, 00133 Rome, Italy; roberto.montanari@uniroma2.it
2. Institute for the Study of Nanostructured Materials, ISMN – CNR, Monterotondo Stazione, 00015 Rome, Italy; Saulius.kaciulis@cnr.it (S.K.); alessio.mezzi@cnr.it (A.M.)
3. Department of Energy, Nuclear Engineering Division, Politecnico di Milano, Piazza L. da Vinci 32, 20133 Milan, Italy; alessandra.fava@uniroma2.it
4. Department of Engineering and Management, University of Padova, Stradella San Nicola 3, 36100 Vicenza, Italy; paolo.ferro@unipd.it
* Correspondence: eleonora.bolli@ismn.cnr.it (E.B.); alessandra.varone@uniroma2.it (A.V.); Tel.: +39-06-90672892 (E.B.); +39-06-72597180 (A.V.)

Received: 4 August 2020; Accepted: 27 August 2020; Published: 29 August 2020

Abstract: The fracture surfaces of a 10.5 wt.% Cr martensitic stainless steel broken in Charpy tests have been investigated through X-ray photoelectron spectroscopy (XPS). The specimens have been examined in two different conditions: as-quenched and heat treated for 10 h at 700 °C. The trends of Fe/Cr ratio vs. test temperature are similar to the sigmoidal curves of absorbed energy and, after both ductile and quasi-cleavage brittle fractures, such ratio is always significantly lower than the nominal value of the steel chemical composition. Cr segregation does not occur on a macroscopic scale but takes place in microscopic zones which represent weaker spots in the steel matrix and a preferred path for moving cracks. Small area (diameter 300 µm) XPS measurements evidenced a higher density of such microscopic zones in the inner part of probes; this is explained by the different diffusion length of Cr atoms in the external and inner parts during quenching from austenitic field which has been calculated through FEM simulations. No significant differences of Cr concentration were observed in fracture surfaces of probes with and without heat treatment. The results highlight how Cr segregation plays a role not only in the intergranular mode of fracture but also in the quasi-cleavage and ductile ones.

Keywords: martensitic stainless steel; Cr segregation; fracture; Charpy test; XPS

1. Introduction

Since the eighties, Cr martensitic steels with controlled impurity contents have drawn the attention of engineers and materials scientists for replacing austenitic stainless steels in structural applications in future nuclear fusion reactors [1–3]. Reduced activation martensitic steels (RAMS) have been developed by substituting alloying elements such as Mo, Nb, Ni, and Co, which cause long-lived transmutation nuclides, with other elements, e.g., W, Ta, and V, leading to relatively short-lived transmutation nuclides. A review of the work done from early stages of RAMS to their more recent qualification for reactor design codes is reported in [4]. A lot of research has been devoted to investigating topics such as activation, swelling, embrittlement, and creep resistance because the microstructural and mechanical stability at high temperature and under neutron irradiation is of utmost importance for this application.

The influence of austenitization temperature on martensitic transformation [5,6] and the effects of tempering on texture evolution [7], micro-strains [8,9], and ductile to brittle transition temperature (DBTT) [10] have been carefully studied by examining different RAMS. One of the critical issues in the use of the martensitic steels is the embrittlement induced by heat treatments because martensite decomposes into a Cr-rich α′ and a Cr-poor α phase with consequent progressive hardening and deterioration of fracture toughness [11]. Such phenomenon depends on the Cr content of the alloy and strengthening increases with the size of α′ zones [12].

Since Cr segregation affects many physical phenomena occurring in Fe-Cr or Fe-Cr-C alloys which have different industrial applications, the physical mechanisms and precursor stages are extensively studied. Li et al. [13] investigated by means of atom probe tomography (APT) the C-Cr co-segregation at grain boundaries and found a concentration periodicity of ~7 nm. Through a cross-correlative precession electron diffraction–atom probe tomography investigation the Cr segregation in a Fe(Cr) nanocrystalline alloy was found to be dependent on grain boundary type [14]. Segregation, precipitation, and phase separation in Fe-Cr systems have been analyzed by Kuronen et al. [15], showing that the precipitation of Cr occurs into isolated pockets in bulk Fe-Cr alloys with Cr content higher than 10 at.%. Mirebeau et al. [16] and Dubiel et al. [17–20] evidenced that short range order (SRO) develops in Fe-Cr alloys following prolonged heat treatments up to ~630 °C with a clustering tendency. To explain the corrosion behavior of Fe-Cr alloys Liu et al. [21] considered the effect of SRO on establishing a percolation network of Cr atoms.

A relevant finding of Mechanical Spectroscopy (MS) investigations on Cr martensitic steels is the presence of C-Cr associates and clusters in as-quenched martensite [22]. Small-angle neutron scattering (SANS) measurements showed that their size is <5 nm [6]. The C-Cr associate distribution changes with quenching rate from austenitic field and evolves following heat treatments, leading in some cases to contiguous Cr-rich and Cr-poor zones, which affect both radiation resistance and fracture behaviour [23–25]. Recently, an analytic study of such point defect structures (C-Cr associates) and of their role on Cr segregation has been carried out through MS experiments [26].

Remarkable differences in fracture mode and DBTT have been observed in samples quenched from austenitic field with slow (150 °C/min) and fast (3600 °C/min) cooling rates, and successively heat treated at 700 °C for increasing time. The samples cooled with the slower rate exhibit a mixed mode of brittle fracture (quasi-cleavage plus inter-crystalline) whereas quasi-cleavage fracture is observed in samples cooled with the faster one. This was explained by the Cr enrichment at grain boundaries occurring in slowly cooled samples and favoured by the specific distribution of C-Cr associates after quenching [27]. This represents an important achievement for better understanding the physical mechanisms governing the embrittlement of Cr martensitic steels, however there are some still open problems. Firstly, it is necessary to assess whether Cr segregation, even to a minor extent, occurs also in samples cooled with fast rate. The second problem is to clarify its role in the process of fracture in both ductile and brittle fields.

Moreover, recent X-ray photoelectron spectroscopy (XPS) analyses carried out on the fracture surfaces evidenced the segregation of Cr in both ductile and brittle (quasi-cleavage) fields [28]. To shed more light on these aspects, the fracture behaviour of a Cr martensitic steel prepared in two different conditions, (1) as-quenched with cooling rate of 3600 °C/min and (2) quenched and annealed at 700 °C for 10 h, has been investigated through Charpy tests. Then, XPS measurements have been carried out on the fracture surfaces of probes broken in ductile and brittle field to assess possible variations of Cr content with respect to the mean value of the alloy.

2. Materials and Methods

The nominal composition of the examined martensitic stainless steel is reported in Table 1.

Table 1. Chemical composition of the investigated Cr martensitic steel (wt.%).

C	Cr	Mo	Ni	Mn	Nb	V	Si	Al	N	P	Fe
0.17	10.50	0.50	0.85	0.60	0.20	0.25	0.32	0.05	0.003	0.005	to balance

According to ASTM A370, standard V-notched probes (55 × 10 × 10 mm^3) for Charpy tests were manufactured from a 10 mm-thick plate. They were treated for 30 min at 1075 °C (austenitic field) then quenched with a cooling rate of 3600 °C/min, measured by a thermocouple put in direct contact with the probe surface. A set of probes were tested in as-quenched condition while another set was heated for 10 h at 700 °C.

The Charpy tests were performed according to the UNI EN ISO 148-1:2016 [29] standard in the temperature range from −100 to +150 °C. The image of a broken probe is displayed in Figure 1 while the absorbed energy vs. test temperature is shown in Figure 2. Each point in the graph is the mean value of five tests and the error bars represent the standard deviation. After fitting experimental data through sigmoidal curves DBTT was determined as the temperature corresponding to (USE + LSE)/2, where USE and LSE are the upper and lower shelf energies, respectively. Table 2 reports the values of DBTT and USE determined from the curves in Figure 2. After the heat treatment DBTT shifts towards lower temperatures, the change is ~40 °C.

Table 2. Ductile to brittle transition temperature (DBTT) and USE values determined from the curves in Figure 2.

Heat Treatment	DBTT (°C)	USE (J)
As-quenched	+18	114
10 h/700 °C	−18	142

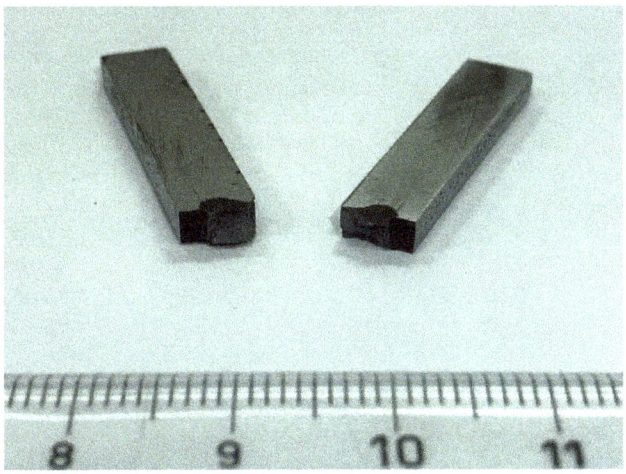

Figure 1. A probe broken in Charpy test (ductile field).

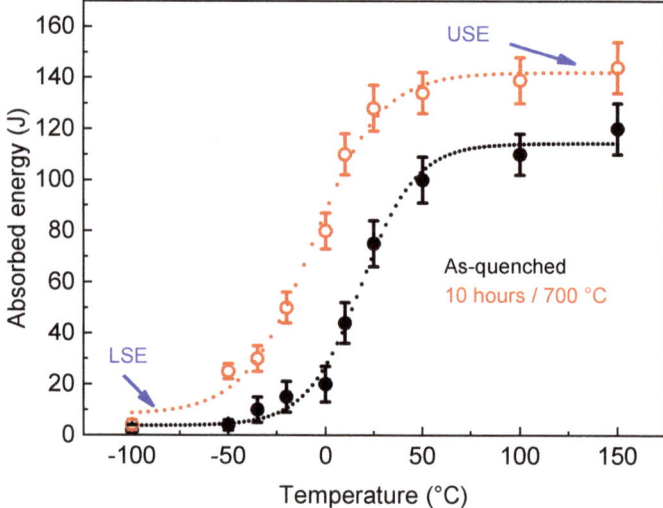

Figure 2. Absorbed energy vs. test temperature of Cr martensitic steel in as-quenched condition and after heat treatment for 10 h at 700 °C.

The material structure after quenching and successive heat treatment has been investigated by scanning electron microscopy (SEM Hitachi SU70, Hitachi, Tokyo, Japan) and X-ray diffraction (XRD). XRD patterns of the most intense reflections have been collected (Philips, Eindhoven, The Netherlands) with the Mo-Kα radiation (λ = 0.071 nm) in step-scanning mode with 2θ steps of 0.005° and counting time of 10 s per step. In order to determine the fracture mode and possible effects of Cr segregation, the surfaces of the probes broken at different temperatures were examined by SEM and EDS microanalysis (Thermo Scientific 4443F, Madison, WI, USA).

The XPS measurements were carried out on the fracture surfaces of the two sets of samples. Because of excessive C contamination, before the analysis each sample was cleaned by the chemical etching at room temperature in a solution of HCl diluted to 12.3% for a duration of 30 s. The acid was then removed by washing the specimens with ultra-pure water in ultrasonic bath. The XPS experiments were performed by using an Escalab 250 Xi (Thermo Fisher Scientific Ltd., East Grinstead, UK) with a monochromatic Al X-ray source (hν = 1486.6 eV) at a spot size of 900 μm. The spectrometer was equipped with a hemispherical analyser and 6-channeltrons as a detector. The fracture surface of every sample was investigated in ultra-high vacuum (UHV), keeping the base pressure in the analysis chamber of about 10^{-10} mbar. The pressure was increased, when the Ar^+ ion gun EX06 was turned on during the XPS depth profiling. The ion gun used for the Ar^+ sputtering was operated at energy of 2 keV and beam current density of 2.5 mA cm^{-2}. XPS regions were acquired at pass energy of 40 eV and standard electromagnetic lens mode, corresponding to ~1 mm in diameter of analyzed sample area. Moreover, multipoint analysis over the fracture surfaces was carried on in small-area lens mode, corresponding to 300 μm in diameter. The binding energy BE = 285.0 eV, corresponding to C1s peak of adventitious carbon, was used for the scale calibration. The spectra were acquired and processed by Avantage v.5 software, where the smart mode background subtraction was applied for quantitative analysis.

A numerical model was developed using Sysweld® code to investigate the thermal gradients within the sample during the imposed rapid cooling. Thermal properties were taken as a function of temperature and phases (Figure 3a). The austenitic to martensitic transformation was modelled using the well-known Koistinen-Marburger equation [30,31] with martensite start temperature set equal to 375 °C. The numerical model, shown in Figure 3b, consisted of 14,000 linear finite elements.

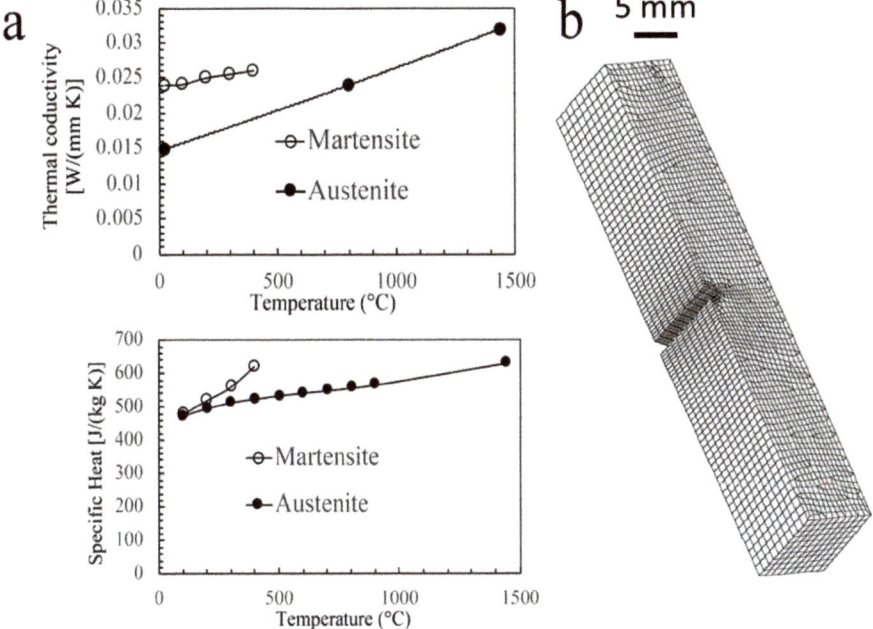

Figure 3. Thermal material properties of the steel investigated (**a**) and 3D numerical model used for the thermal analysis (**b**).

The temperature at nodes belonging to the external surface was made to vary from 1075 °C to room temperature with a constant cooling rate of 3600 °C/min (boundary condition).

3. Results and Discussion

It is well known that C and impurities like P are site competitors, thus the free C atoms tend to suppress P segregation at grain boundaries and consequently intergranular embrittlement. Since Cr or other carbide-forming elements decrease the concentration of free C in the steel matrix, it is reasonable to expect high impurity grain boundary segregation in an alloy with Cr content > 11 wt.%. In the examined steel, P content is very low (0.005 wt.%) to avoid specific embrittlement; the P rich χ-phase was found to nucleate during proton irradiation at pre-existing NbC precipitates [32], however P segregation after heat treatments at 700 °C is not reported in literature. Therefore, the attention of present work is focused on Cr segregation.

The microstructural evolution induced by heat treatments is displayed in Figure 4. After quenching, the steel is fully martensitic and exhibits a typical martensitic structure consisting of laths organized in packets; each prior austenitic grain (PAG) contains several packets. After the heat treatments, the laths disappear, $M_{23}C_6$ (M = Cr, Fe) carbides form decorating PAGs and the interfaces between previous laths. The mean chemical composition (wt.%) of $M_{23}C_6$ carbides is C 6%, Cr 65%, and Fe 29%. Since the carbide precipitation is substantially completed after 2 h at 700 °C, no remarkable difference is observed between the samples treated for 10 h. The Cr profiles in the images of Figure 4 do not show a specific trend but only fluctuations from point to point. Such Cr fluctuations are of the order of 7–8 wt.%.

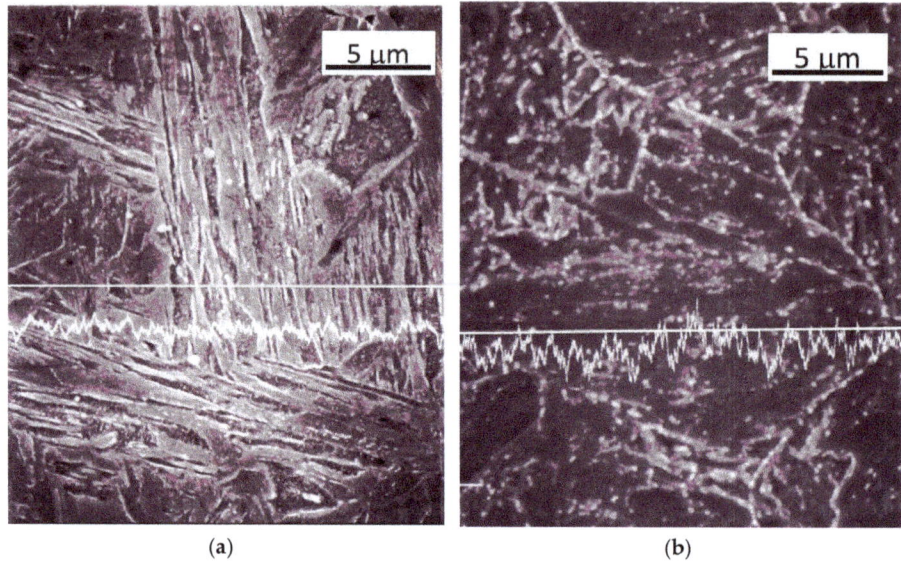

Figure 4. Structure of the steel as-quenched (**a**) and after the heat treatment at 700 °C for 10 h (**b**).

Table 3 reports the line breadths β(2θ) of the most intense XRD reflections, namely {110}, {200} and {211}. In general, the β(2θ) is progressively decreasing after the heat treatments due to the recovery of dislocation structures forming during the martensitic transformation consequent to the quenching from austenitic field.

Table 3. Line breadth β(2θ) of the most intense X-ray diffraction (XRD) reflections.

Heat Treatment	β(2θ)$_{110}$	β(2θ)$_{200}$	β(2θ)$_{211}$
As-quenched	0.28	0.250	0.210
10 h at 700 °C	0.21	0.200	0.150

Figure 5 shows the fracture surfaces of the probes broken in Charpy tests in brittle and ductile field. The surfaces of the probes broken in brittle field exhibit the typical morphological features of quasi-cleavage fracture mode consisting of flat or slightly concave facets that arise from individual micro-cracks. They form independently and propagate through the material until coalesce. Tear ridges are observed in the zones, where the rupture of metal ligaments between different micro-cracks occurs leading to their coalescence (see the sketch in Figure 6). The fine steps inside each facet form when the propagating crack crosses groups of dislocations.

In the fracture surfaces of the samples heated at 700 °C, several carbides are present and the zones, where the detachment of metal from carbides occurs, act as preferred nucleation sites for micro-cracks.

In the case of the ductile fractures, the dimples are the main characteristic. After heat treatment the dimple size shifts to larger dimensions but the morphology does not change; in addition, cracked $M_{23}C_6$ carbides (indicated by arrows in Figure 4) are observed inside the dimples.

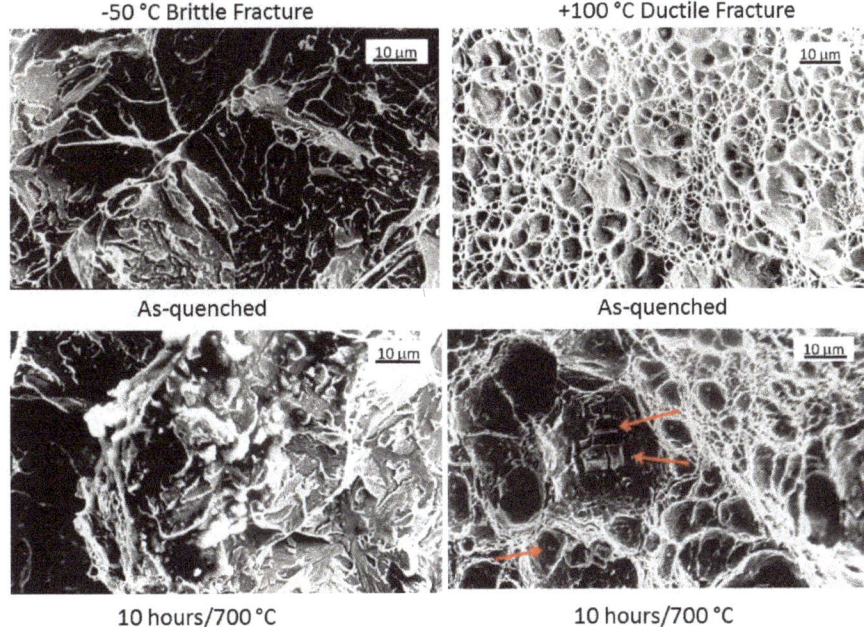

Figure 5. Fracture surfaces of the steel probes broken in Charpy tests in brittle (−50 °C) and ductile field (+ 100 °C).

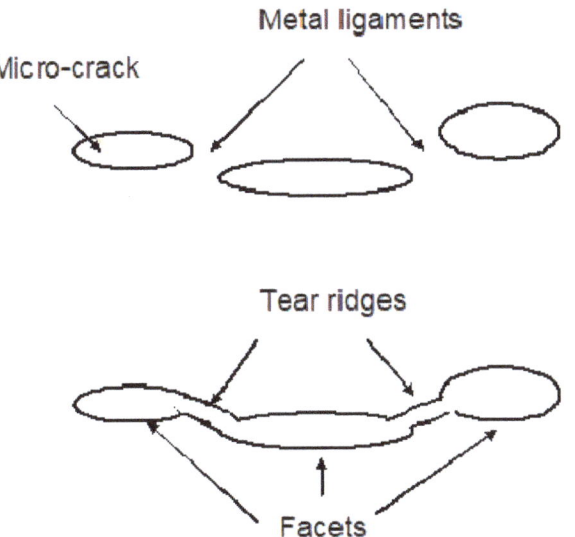

Figure 6. Schematic view of the coalescence process of micro-cracks in quasi-cleavage fracture mode.

The fracture surfaces of the two sets of samples have been investigated by XPS measurements. The spectra of whole Fe 2p and Cr 2p regions were acquired, but only the principal $2p_{3/2}$ peaks were taken into account for the qualitative and quantitative analysis in order to simplify the peak fitting procedure and to increase the accuracy of quantification. Figure 7 shows the Fe $2p_{3/2}$ and Cr $2p_{3/2}$

peaks of the XPS spectra measured on the fracture surfaces of as-quenched steel in both brittle (a,b) and ductile fields (c,d).

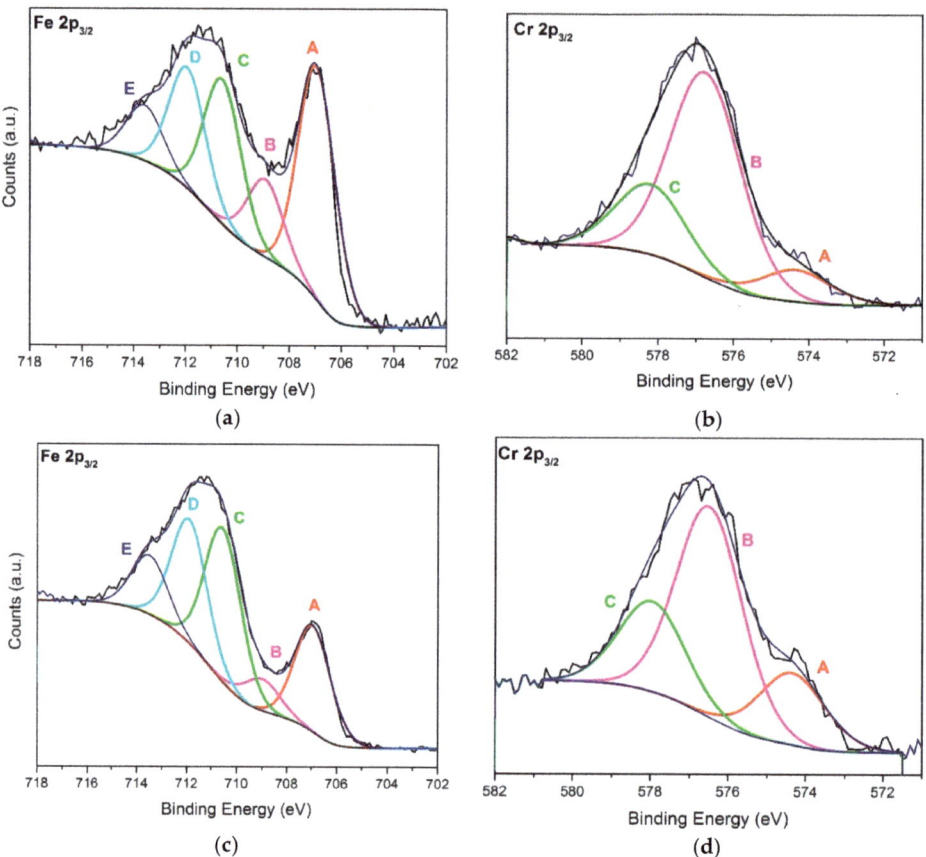

Figure 7. Peak fitting of Fe 2p$_{3/2}$ and Cr 2p$_{3/2}$ spectra of as-quenched samples broken in brittle (−100 °C) field (**a**,**b**) and ductile (+150 °C) field (**c**,**d**).

The attribution of oxidation states for the components of Cr and Fe peaks was carried out after the "smart" background subtraction. The components of Fe 2p$_{3/2}$ spectra (see Figure 7a,c) were the following: the first peak A at BE = 707.0 eV corresponding to metallic Fe^0, peak B at BE = 708.9 eV corresponding to oxidized iron state Fe^{2+} and two other components C at BE = 710.6 eV and D at BE = 711.9 eV corresponding to iron states Fe^{3+} in oxide and hydroxide, respectively [33,34]. The last fitted component E at BE = 713.6 eV is a satellite peak, typical for the Fe oxides. Additionally, the Cr 2p$_{3/2}$ spectra (see Figure 7b,d) had a metallic component A at BE = 574.3 eV and two components of Cr^{3+} states in oxide and hydroxide at BE = 576.8 eV (B) and BE = 578.2 eV (C), respectively [35]. All the components of Fe 2p$_{3/2}$ and Cr 2p$_{3/2}$ spectra, the quantitative weight percentage and respective chemical states are reported in Tables 4 and 5.

Table 4. Binding energy, X-ray photoelectron spectroscopy (XPS) quantification and chemical states of Fe and Cr of the samples broken in brittle field.

Peak	BE (eV)	As-Quenched Wt.% (T_{charpy}: −100 °C)	10 h Wt.% (T_{charpy}: −100 °C)	State
$Fe2p_{3/2}$–A	707.0	24.0	31.7	Fe^0
$Fe2p_{3/2}$–B	708.9	12.5	10.2	Fe^{+2}
$Fe2p_{3/2}$–C	710.6	5.7	9.0	Fe^{+3}
$Fe2p_{3/2}$–D	711.9	8.0	6.8	FeOOH
$Fe2p_{3/2}$–E	713.6	14.9	4.3	Satellite
Fe_{total}	-	65.1	62.0	-
$Cr2p_{3/2}$–A	574.3	3.8	8.1	Cr^0
$Cr2p_{3/2}$–B	576.8	23.1	22.1	Cr(III) ox
$Cr2p_{3/2}$–C	578.2	8.0	7.8	Cr(III) hydrox
Cr_{total}	-	34.9	38.0	-

Table 5. Binding energy, XPS quantification, and chemical states of Fe and Cr of the samples broken in ductile field.

Peak	BE (eV)	As-Quenched Wt.% (T_{charpy}: +100 °C)	10 h Wt.% (T_{charpy}: +100 °C)	State
$Fe2p_{3/2}$–A	707.0	18.1	10.8	Fe^0
$Fe2p_{3/2}$–B	708.9	5.4	1.7	Fe^{+2}
$Fe2p_{3/2}$–C	710.6	26.1	31.3	Fe^{+3}
$Fe2p_{3/2}$–D	711.9	21.1	25.3	FeOOH
$Fe2p_{3/2}$–E	713.6	10.0	11.0	Satellite
Fe_{total}	-	80.0	80.1	-
$Cr2p_{3/2}$–A	574.3	3.7	1.5	Cr^0
$Cr2p_{3/2}$–B	576.8	10.9	16.7	Cr(III) ox
$Cr2p_{3/2}$–C	578.2	5.7	1.7	Cr(III) hydrox
Cr_{total}	-	20.0	19.9	-

The same chemical states of Fe and Cr were present in all the fracture surfaces analysed, but the relative intensity of the metallic component with respect to oxide was changing. The intensity of metal and oxide components was very variable: these changes were found not only in different samples but also on different points of the same sample surface. Therefore, the overlayer of segregated Cr on the fracture surface layer is quite thin and not always homogeneously distributed. This result was visible from the comparison of the intensity between the $Fe2p_{3/2}$ components. In fact, in some specific surface areas, where the content of Cr was higher, the metallic Fe peak at BE = 707.0 eV had the same intensity of oxide component at BE = 710.6 eV. In the cases where the amount of Cr was lower, the metallic Fe^0 component was less intense than the oxidized one (see Figure 7c,d). Therefore, it could be assumed that metallic Fe^0 on the surface is covered by a thin Cr film. Since the XPS measurements are extremely sensitive to the surface, the Cr overlayer must be quite thin (less than about 10 nm) for the registration of Fe 2p signal from metallic Fe^0.

This hypothesis was also confirmed by the results of XPS depth profiles carried out on a surface area of 1.5 × 1.5 mm^2 with Ar^+ sputtering cycles of 30 s at ion energy of 2 keV. From these profiles (Figure 8) it was estimated that the Cr-rich overlayer has a mean thickness of few nanometers in all the samples, independently on the test temperature or treatment time. Just a very short Ar^+ sputtering was enough for the complete removal of segregated Cr. In fact, after about 70–80 s of ion sputtering, the Cr signal is strongly reduced for any type of analysed fracture surfaces. From these results, it was possible to estimate the thickness of Cr overlayer. By using the calibrated sputtering rate of 0.17 nm/s, it was calculated that after 70–80 s of sputtering an overlayer of approximately 12–13 nm was removed from the surface. Unfortunately, this time-to-depth conversion is not very accurate, because it refers to ideal conditions, where the sample has a flat surface, whereas the steel fracture surfaces, especially those obtained in ductile field, were very irregular with the result of a shadowed sputtering effect, i.e., a non-uniform sputtering of the fracture surface [36]. For this reason, it is more correct to report the depth profiles in time scale, remembering that the thickness of Cr overlayer is over-estimated in the above calculation.

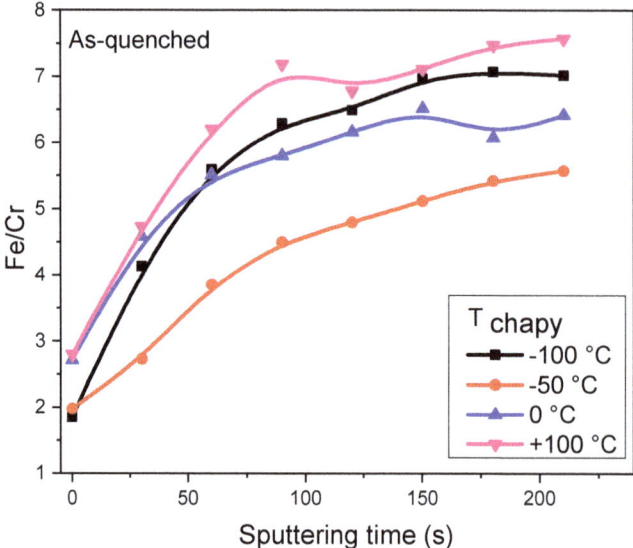

Figure 8. XPS depth profiles of Fe/Cr ratio for as-quenched probes broken in Charpy tests at different temperatures.

To determine the Cr distribution, small-area (diameter of 300 µm) XPS line scans have been carried out across the fracture surfaces of probes broken in ductile (+100 °C) and brittle (−50 and −100 °C) fields. As shown in Figure 9a–c displaying the content (wt.%) of Fe and Cr in different positions, the Cr distribution is much more homogeneous in the probes broken in ductile than in brittle field. It is evident that a strong Cr segregation is present at the centre of the brittle fracture surfaces (black line), of as-quenched and heat treated probes, whereas in the case of ductile fractures (red line) the Cr content is almost constant through the whole surface.

From the quantitative analysis of Fe $2p_{3/2}$ and Cr $2p_{3/2}$ peaks, it was observed an excess of Cr on the fracture surface of all the samples. This phenomenon is much stronger for the fractures obtained in brittle field, where about 40 wt.% of Cr was observed, however Cr is always higher than 20 wt.% also in ductile field, namely well above the value (10.5 wt.%) of the steel nominal composition. These results are different from the Cr line scans obtained by EDS and reported in Figure 4, because the analysis depths of the two techniques are quite different. The maximum information depth of XPS is about 10 nm whereas in EDS it is in the micrometric scale and representative of the bulk value.

To verify whether the Cr enrichment evidenced by line scans of Figure 9a–c, is a specific feature of the fracture paths or, on the contrary, it is somehow connected to a macro-segregation phenomenon of the probes, the tests were also carried out under the same conditions on 6 different points of the flat surface of a probe cross-section after mechanical polishing (see Figure 9c). The average content of Cr was calculated to be of 10.6 ± 0.3 wt.%, corresponding to an experimental error less than 5% and, consequently, less than 10% for what concerns the Fe/Cr ratio. From the data in Figure 9c, it is evident that there is no macro-segregation because the contents of Fe and Cr do not depend on the position, are nearly constant, and correspond to the nominal values of the steel composition. So, these results showed that the XPS data are extremely repeatable, consequently, the calculated values of the Fe/Cr ratio, were in any case lower than the nominal ratio, after adding the experimental error. Therefore, the profiles in Figure 9a,b are specific of the fracture paths which advance through the material along the way of minor resistance, namely through the zones with higher Cr content.

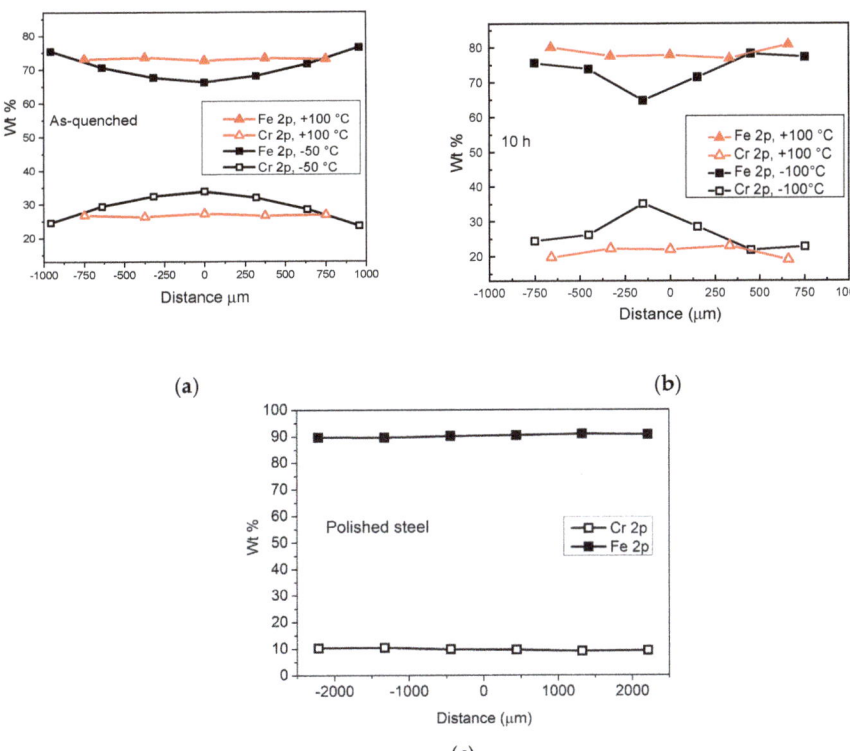

Figure 9. Small-area XPS line scans across the fracture surfaces of probes broken in brittle and ductile fields: (**a**) as-quenched and (**b**) treated at 700 °C for 10 h. The indicated distance is taken from the fracture centre. For comparison, the scan of the cross-section of an as-quenched probe after mechanical polishing is shown in (**c**).

In order to deepen the Cr segregation phenomenon, the thermal gradients within the probe during cooling were determined via numerical simulation. For example, Figure 10 shows the profiles of temperature through a Charpy probe after a given time of cooling (t = 1.39 min) as well as the corresponding distribution of martensite volume fraction. The inner part of the probe experiences a slower cooling than the surface thus the martensitic transformation starts at the surface and then moves to the inner part of the probe. In Figure 10b, the external part consists of martensite (red color), the inner part of austenite (blue color), while in the middle there is the presence of both the phases in different fractions depending on the distance from the surface. At room temperature the predicted microstructure is fully martensitic as in the real sample.

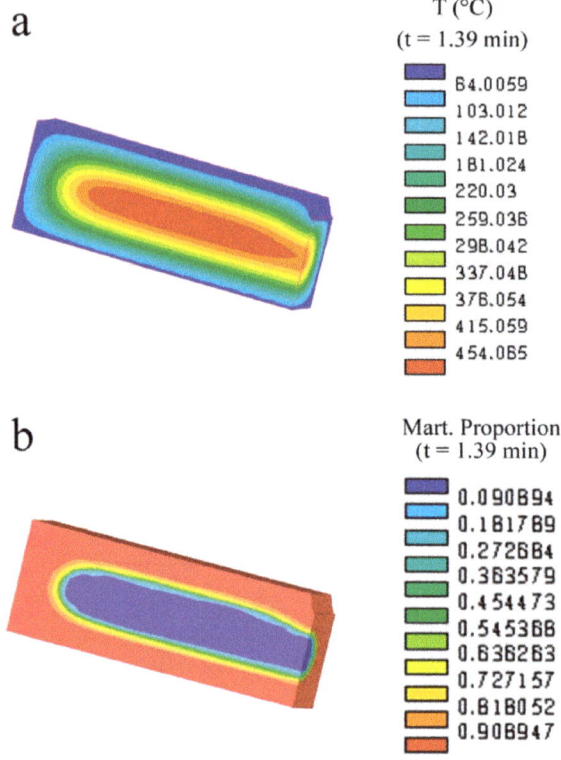

Figure 10. Calculated temperature (**a**) and martensite proportion (**b**) distribution at 1.39 min during cooling.

The thermal histories captured by two virtual probes located in the center (point A) and on the surface (point B) of the cross section in correspondence of the notch are shown in Figure 11. The temperature inside the specimen (point A) during cooling is used to estimate the Cr diffusion distances close to the center of fracture surface.

In the conditions of present experiments, the random walk (*RW*) of C and Cr atoms at the surface and in the internal part of Charpy probes was calculated vs. time on the basis of the trends reported in Figure 11. The calculation was made only for the austenitic phase because RW is negligible after the martensitic transformation at 375 °C. This permits also to neglect the Cr partitioning between austenite and martensite occurring in steels during isothermal treatments (e.g., see [37]).

RW for the temperature *T* and time t is given by:

$$RW = (6Dt)^{1/2} \tag{1}$$

where *D* is the diffusion coefficient. The diffusion coefficients of *C* and *Cr* in austenite were determined according to the following expressions:

$$D_C = 1.0 \times 10^{-5} \exp\left(\frac{-32400}{RT}\right) (m^2 \ s^{-1}) \tag{2}$$

$$D_{Cr} = 1.08 \times 10^3 \exp\left(\frac{-69700}{RT}\right) (m^2 \ s^{-1}) \tag{3}$$

being R the gas constant (= 1.987 [cal mol^{-1} K^{-1}]). The RW values of C and Cr in points A and B plotted in Figure 12a,b were determined by integrating Equation (1) with time steps dt of 0.06 s.

Of course, RW of C is always higher than that of Cr, however the most interesting result is the significant difference for both the elements between external and internal parts. In fact, the internal part of Charpy probes undergoes a slower cooling which allows a longer diffusion path of C and Cr atoms. Several experimental [15,18–21] and simulation [15,20] works give clear evidence of the clustering tendency in Fe-Cr alloys which decreases as temperature increases, however MS measurements [5] and Monte Carlo simulations [24] showed that some Cr atoms aggregation occurs also in austenitic field, in particular C-Cr associates [22,26] act as preferred sites for the clustering of Cr atoms. It is evident that higher RW values involve favorable conditions for Cr atoms aggregation. As shown by Figure 9c, the formation of Cr enriched zones does not take place on a macroscopic scale otherwise it would be detected also on the polished surface of the probes but only on a microscopic scale.

In order to highlight the effects of Cr clustering on impact behaviour, the ratio Fe/Cr of the mean values (wt.%) measured on the fracture surface of all the samples has been calculated. From the nominal composition of steel, this ratio is 8.2 in the bulk material, whereas its value is noticeably lower for all the fracture surfaces, as shown by the plots in Figure 13.

The graphs of Fe/Cr ratio vs. test temperature are somehow similar to the sigmoidal curves of absorbed energy displayed in Figure 2. For both the probe sets, the surfaces originated from brittle fractures exhibit a higher Cr content than the ductile ones, however the Fe/Cr ratio is always rather far from the value corresponding to the chemical composition of the steel. The fracture surfaces are always enriched in Cr and this means that the microscopic Cr enriched zones represent a preferred path for cracks in both modes of fracture (brittle and ductile).

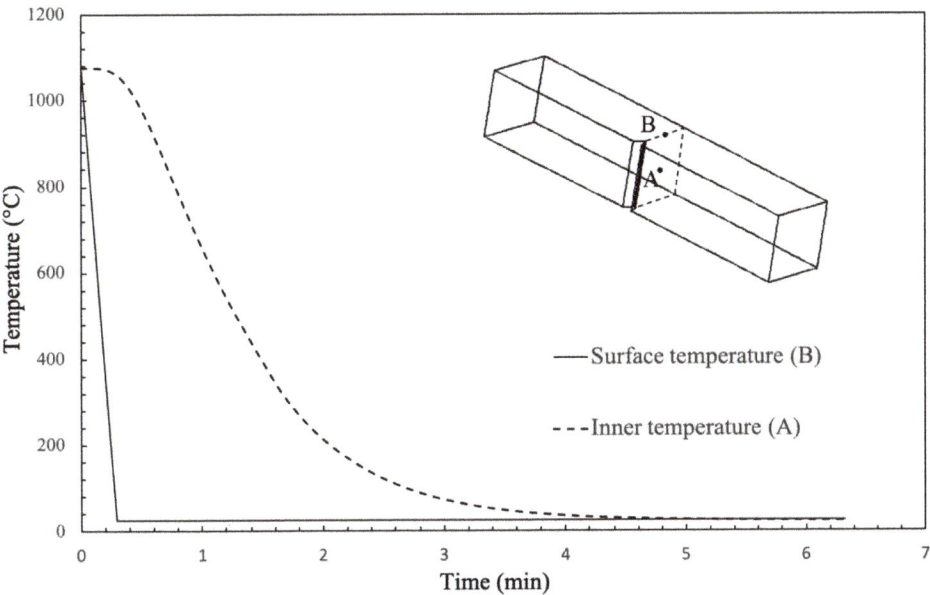

Figure 11. Calculated temperature histories at two points (A and B) of the Charpy specimen.

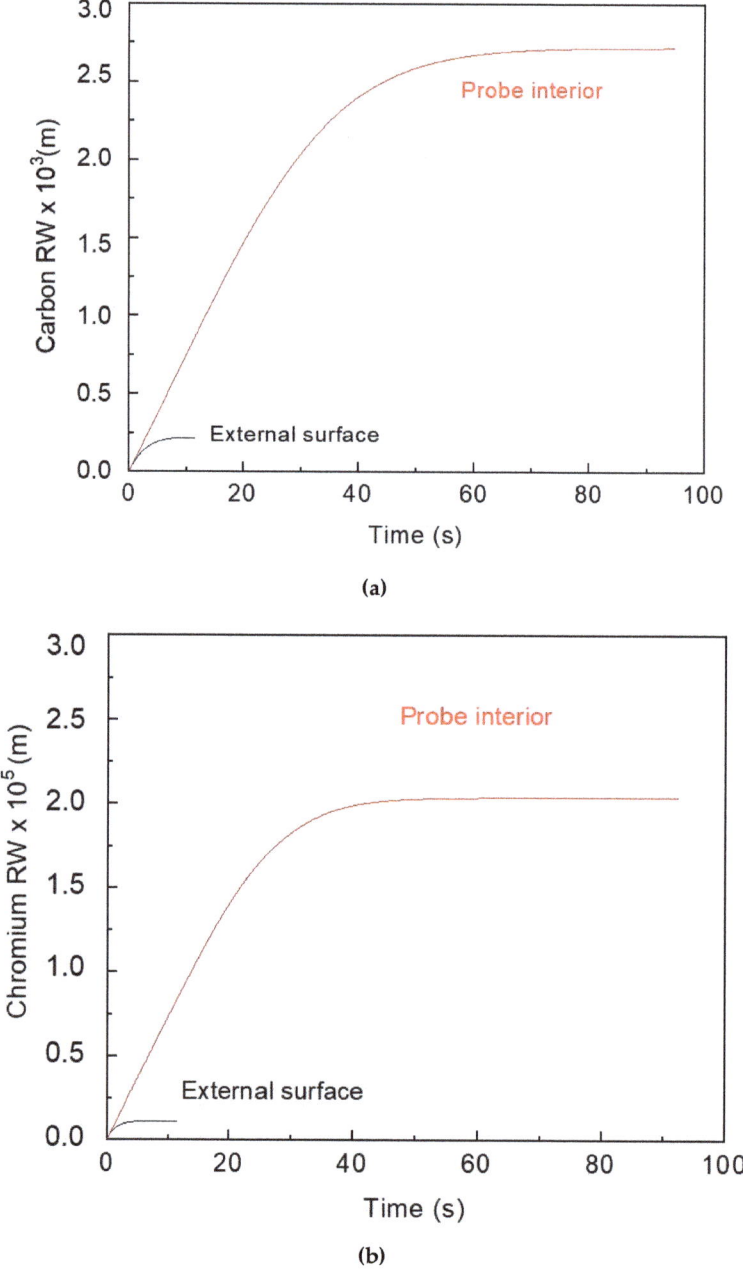

Figure 12. Random walk (*RW*) of C (**a**) and Cr (**b**) atoms vs. time at the surface and in the internal part of Charpy probes calculated on the basis of the trends reported in Figure 11.

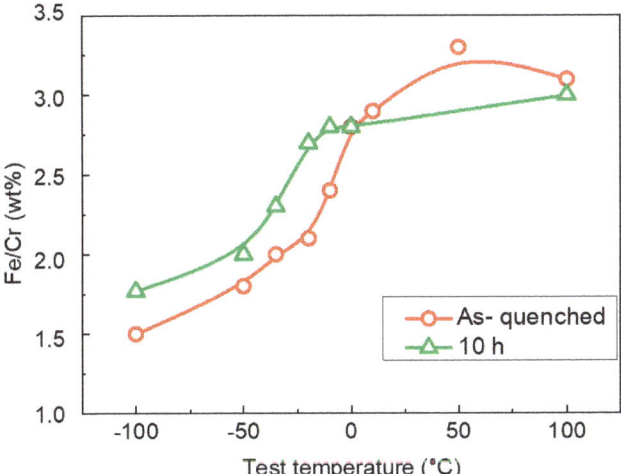

Figure 13. Fe/Cr (wt.%) vs. test temperature of Cr martensitic steel in as-quenched condition and after the heat treatment for 10 at 700 °C.

Line scans (Figure 9) and mean Fe/Cr values (Figure 13) do not show relevant difference of Cr concentration in the surfaces resulting from ductile fractures of probes with and without heat treatment, while a little difference is observed in brittle field. In Fe-Cr alloys, the Mössbauer measurements [20] indicate a decreasing trend of short-range ordering (SRO) parameter as temperature increases, however there is still a tendency to Cr clustering up to 700 °C. Therefore, the heat treatment (10 h at 700 °C) is not suitable to achieve the homogeneous Cr distribution in the steel matrix. A part of Cr atoms (~2.5 wt.%) [30] forms carbides (see Figure 3) but remaining Cr atoms are not uniformly distributed.

Previous works [10] on the same steel slowly cooled from austenitic field (150 °C/min) showed that a mixed mode of fracture (quasi-cleavage plus inter-crystalline) occurs and EDS measurements evidenced Cr segregation in the areas of inter-crystalline fracture. This is in agreement with the theoretical work of Seah [38] and with experimental investigations on steels of similar composition [39] and more generally on Fe-Cr alloys [40]. The embrittlement due to grain boundary segregation is the sum of effects due to bond-breaking, chemical interactions, and atomic size effects [41]. In the conditions of faster cooling rate (3600 °C/min) examined here, the steel does not exhibit inter-crystalline fracture mode, however XPS results indicate that Cr segregation plays a role also in other modes of fracture including quasi-cleavage and ductile fractures.

No papers report specific XPS studies on the fracture surfaces of this material and, more in general, the literature is lacking in publications dealing with micro-chemical analyses on Cr martensitic steels. In the past, Auger electron spectroscopy (e.g., see [42–44]) has been used for studying high temperature embrittlement but the examined materials had a much higher P content than the steel examined here and the attention was focused on the role of C and Cr in determining the P content in grain boundaries. More recently, an investigation carried out by means of Scanning Auger Microscopy (SAM) on the fracture mode of turbine blades before and after service life shows that there is change in brittle fracture mode from intergranular to transgranular induced by a Cr redistribution from grain boundaries towards grain interior [44]. The mechanisms through which Cr segregation affects quasi-cleavage and ductile fracture modes are not yet completely clear and the topic deserves further investigation, therefore experiments are underway on sets of probes treated at increasing time at 700 °C.

4. Conclusions

XPS measurements have been carried out on the fracture surfaces of a Cr martensitic stainless steel in as-quenched condition and after a heat treatment of 10 h at 700 °C. The results can be summarized as follows.

1. The mean Fe/Cr ratio determined on the fracture surfaces of probes broken in both ductile and brittle fields is always significantly lower than the value corresponding to the steel nominal composition.
2. Small-area measurements revealed that the Fe/Cr ratio is not constant across the surface and is lower in the inner part of the probe. FEM simulations show that this is due to a slower cooling rate in the inner part of Charpy probes that allows longer random walk of diffusing atoms.
3. The effect is observed in fractured probes but not in cross-sections after mechanical polishing, thus Cr segregation does not occur on macroscopic scale.
4. The Cr enrichment on the fracture surfaces indicates that the crack path preferentially follows the zones with Cr segregation.
5. Relevant differences of Cr concentration in fracture surfaces of probes with and without heat treatment were not observed.

Experiments are underway on sets of the probes treated for increasing time at 700 °C in order to understand the specific mechanisms relating Cr segregation and quasi-cleavage and ductile fractures.

Author Contributions: Conceptualization, E.B., A.F., P.F., S.K., A.M., R.M. and A.V.; Investigation, E.B., A.F., P.F., S.K., A.M., R.M. and A.V.; Validation, E.B., A.F., P.F., S.K., A.M., R.M. and A.V.; Writing, R.M., S.K. and E.B. All authors have read and agreed to the published version of the manuscript.

Funding: This work has been carried out within the framework of the EUROfusion Consortium and has received funding from the Euratom research and training programme 2014–2018 and 2019–2020 under Grant Agreement No. 633053. The views and opinions expressed herein do not necessarily reflect those of the European Commission.

Acknowledgments: The authors are grateful to Piero Plini and Benedetto Iacovone of Department of Industrial Engineering–University of Rome "Tor Vergata" for the assistance in sample preparation.

Conflicts of Interest: The authors declare no conflict of interest.

References

1. Mansur, L.K.; Coghlan, W.A. Mechanisms of helium interaction with radiation effects in metals and alloys: A review. *J. Nucl. Mater.* **1983**, *119*, 1–25. [CrossRef]
2. Harrelson, K.J.; Rou, S.H.; Wilcox, R.C. Impurity element effects on the toughness of 9Cr-1Mo steel. *J. Nucl. Mater.* **1986**, *141–143*, 508–512. [CrossRef]
3. Coppola, R.; Gondi, P.; Montanari, R.; Veniali, F. Structure evolution during heat treatments of 12% Cr martensitic steel for NET. *J. Nucl. Mater.* **1988**, *155–157*, 616–619. [CrossRef]
4. Tavassoli, A.-A.F.; Diegele, E.; Lindau, R.; Luzginova, N.; Tanigawa, H. Current status and recent research achievements in ferritic/martensitic steels. *J. Nucl. Mater.* **2014**, *455*, 269–276. [CrossRef]
5. Gondi, P.; Montanari, R.; Sili, A. Effects of high temperature treatments on martensitic transformation in MANET steel. *Z. Für Metallkd.* **1994**, *85*, 664–669.
6. Albertini, G.; Ceretti, M.; Coppola, R.; Fiori, F.; Gondi, P.; Montanari, R. Small-angle neutron scattering of C-Cr elementary aggregates in a martensitic steel for fusion reactor technology. *Physica B* **1995**, *213–214*, 812–814. [CrossRef]
7. Brokmeier, H.G.; Coppola, R.; Montanari, R.; Rustichelli, F. Neutron diffraction study of the crystalline texture in a martensitic steel for fusion reactor technology. *Physica B* **1995**, *213–214*, 809–811. [CrossRef]
8. Brunelli, L.; Gondi, P.; Montanari, R.; Coppola, R. Internal strains after recovery of hardness in tempered martensitic steels for fusion reactors. *J. Nucl. Mater.* **1991**, *179–181*, 675. [CrossRef]
9. Coppola, R.; Lukas, P.; Montanari, R.; Rustichelli, F.; Vrana, M. X-ray and neutron line broadening measurements in a martensitic steel for fusion technology. *Mater. Lett.* **1995**, *22*, 17. [CrossRef]

10. Gondi, P.; Montanari, R.; Sili, A.; Tata, M.E. Effects of thermal treatments on the ductile to brittle transition of MANET steel. *J. Nucl. Mater.* **1996**, *233–237*, 248–252. [CrossRef]
11. Hedströma, P.; Baghsheikhia, S.; Liu, P.; Odqvist, J. A phase-field and electron microscopy study of phase separation in Fe-Cr alloys. *J. Mater. Sci. Eng. A* **2012**, *534*, 552–556. [CrossRef]
12. Chen, D.; Kimura, A.; Han, W. Correlation of Fe/Cr phase decomposition process and age-hardening in Fe-15Cr ferritic alloys. *J. Nucl. Mater.* **2014**, *455*, 436–439. [CrossRef]
13. Li, H.; Xia, S.; Zhou, B.; Liu, W. C-Cr segregation at grain boundary before the carbide nucleation in Alloy 690. *Mater. Charact.* **2012**, *66*, 68–74. [CrossRef]
14. Zhou, X.; Yu, X.; Kaub, T.; Martens, R.L.; Thompson, G.B. Grain Boundary Specific Segregation in Nanocrystalline Fe (Cr). *Nat. Sci. Rep.* **2016**, *6*, 1–14. [CrossRef]
15. Kuronen, A.; Granroth, S.; Heinonen, M.H.; Perälä, R.E.; Kilpi, T.; Laukkanen, P.; Lång, J.; Dahl, J.; Punkkinen, M.P.J.; Kokko, K.; et al. Segregation, precipitation, and α-α phase separation in Fe-Cr alloys. *Phys. Rev. B* **2015**, *92*, 1–16. [CrossRef]
16. Mirebeau, I.; Parette, G. Neutron Study of The Short Range Order Inversion in Fe1-x Crx. *Phys. Rev. B* **2010**, *82*, 1–5. [CrossRef]
17. Dubiel, S.M.; Cieslak, J. Short-Range Order in Iron-Rich Fe-Cr Alloys as Revealed by Mössbauer Spectroscopy. *Phys. Rev. B* **2011**, *83*, 1–4. [CrossRef]
18. Dubiel, S.M.; Cieslak, J. Effect of Thermal Treatment on the Short-Range Order in Fe-Cr Alloys. *Mater. Lett.* **2013**, *107*, 86–89. [CrossRef]
19. Dubiel, S.M.; Cieslak, J.; Zukrowski, J. Distribution of Cr Atoms in The Surface Zone of Fe-Rich Fe-Cr Alloys Quenched into Various Media: Mössbauer Spectroscopic Study. *Appl. Surf. Sci.* **2015**, *359*, 526–532. [CrossRef]
20. Idczak, R.; Konieczny, R. Temperature dependence of the short-range order parameter for $Fe_{0.90}Cr_{0.10}$ and $Fe_{0.88}Cr_{0.12}$ alloys. *Nukleonika* **2015**, *60*, 35–38. [CrossRef]
21. Liu, M.; Aiello, A.; Xie, Y.; Sieradzki, K. The Effect of Short-Range Order on Passivation of Fe-Cr Alloys. *J. Electrochem. Soc.* **2018**, *165*, C830–C834. [CrossRef]
22. Gondi, P.; Montanari, R. On the Cr distribution in MANET steel. *Phys. Status Solidi A* **1992**, *131*, 465–480. [CrossRef]
23. Gondi, P.; Montanari, R. Q^{-1} spectra connected with C under solute atom interaction. *J. Alloys Compd.* **1994**, *211-212*, 33. [CrossRef]
24. Coppola, R.; Gondi, P.; Montanari, R. Effects of C-Cr elementary aggregates on the properties of the MANET steel. *J. Nucl. Mater.* **1993**, *206*, 360–362. [CrossRef]
25. Gondi, P.; Montanari, R.; Sili, A.; Coppola, R. Solute Cr atom distribution and fracture behaviour of MANET steel. *J. Nucl. Mater.* **1994**, *212–215*, 564–568. [CrossRef]
26. Fava, A.; Montanari, R.; Varone, A. Mechanical spectroscopy investigation of point defects driven phenomena in a Cr martensitic steel. *Metals* **2018**, *8*, 870. [CrossRef]
27. Bolli, E.; Fava, A.; Kaciulis, S.; Mezzi, A.; Montanari, R.; Varone, A. XPS study of Cr segregation in a martensitic stainless steel. *Surf. Interface Anal.* **2020**, 1–4. [CrossRef]
28. Xue, M.; Wang, S.; Wu, K.; Guo, J.; Guo, Q. Surface structural evolution in iron oxide thin films. *Langmuir* **2011**, *27*, 11–14. [CrossRef]
29. UNI EN ISO 148-1:2016 The International Organization for Standardization. *Metallic Materials-Charpy Pendulum Impact Test (www.iso.org/obp/ui/#iso:std:iso:148:-3:ed-3:v1:en)*; ISO: Geneva, Switzerland, 2016.
30. Koistinen, D.P.; Marburger, R.E. A general equation prescribing extent of austenite-martensite transformation in pure iron-carbon alloys and carbon steels. *Acta Metall.* **1959**, *7*, 59–68. [CrossRef]
31. Ferro, P.; Bonollo, F.; Berto, F.; Montanari, R. Numerical modelling of residual stress redistribution induced by TIG-dressing. *Frattura Integrità Strutt.* **2019**, *47*, 221–230. [CrossRef]
32. Jung, P.; Klein, H. Segregation in DIN 1.4914 martensitic stainless steel under proton irradiation. *J. Nucl. Mater.* **1991**, *182*, 1–5. [CrossRef]
33. Lin, T.-C.; Seshadri, G.; Kelber, J.A. A consistent method for quantitative XPS peak analysis of thin oxide films on clean polycrystalline iron surfaces. *Appl. Surf. Sci.* **1997**, *119*, 83–92. [CrossRef]
34. Biesinger, M.C.; Payne, B.P.; Grosvenor, A.P.; Lau, L.W.M.; Gerson, A.R.; Smart, R.S.C. Resolving surface chemical states in XPS analysis of first row transition metals, oxides and hydroxides: Cr, Mn, Fe, Co and Ni. *Appl. Surf. Sci.* **2011**, *257*, 2717–2730. [CrossRef]

35. Hofmann, S. Depth Profiling in AES and XPS. In *Practical Surface Analysis*; Briggs, D., Seah, M.P.J., Eds.; Wiley and Sons: Chichester, UK, 1990; pp. 143–199.
36. De Sanctis, M.; Valentini, R.; Lovicu, G.F.; Dimatteo, A.; Migliaccio, U.; Montanari, R.; Pietrangeli, E. Microstructural features affecting tempering behaviour of 16Cr-5Ni supermartensitic steel. *Metall. Mater. Trans. A* **2015**, *46*, 1878–1887. [CrossRef]
37. Seah, M.P. Adsorption-induced interface decohesion. *Acta Metall.* **1980**, *28*, 955–962. [CrossRef]
38. Schäublin, R.; Spätig, P.; Victoria, M. Chemical segregation behavior of the low activation ferritic/martensitic steel F82H. *J. Nucl. Mater.* **1998**, *258–263*, 1350–1355. [CrossRef]
39. Saraf, L.V.; Lea, A.S.; Wang, C.M.; Dohnalkova, A.; Arey, B.W. Chromium Segregation at the Grain Boundaries in Ni-Fe-Cr Alloys. *Microsc. Microanal.* **2010**, *16*, 690–691. [CrossRef]
40. Gibson, M.A.; Schuh, C.A. A survey of ab-initio calculations shows that segregation-induced grain boundary embrittlement is predicted by bond-breaking arguments. *Scr. Mater.* **2016**, *113*, 55–58. [CrossRef]
41. Lemble, P.H.; Pineau, A.; Castagne, J.L.; Dumoulin, P. Temper embrittlement in 12%Cr martensitic steel. *Met. Sci.* **1979**, *13*, 496–502. [CrossRef]
42. Prabhu Gaunkar, G.V.; Huntz, A.M.; Lacombe, P. Role of carbon in embrittlement phenomena of tempered martensitic 12%–0.15% C steel. *Met. Sci.* **1980**, *14*, 241–252. [CrossRef]
43. Lei, T.C.; Sun, J.; Tang, C.H.; Lei, M. Precipitation-segregation mechanism for high temperature temper embrittlement of steels revealed by Auger electron spectroscopy and internal friction measurements. *Mater. Sci. Technol.* **1990**, *6*, 124–133. [CrossRef]
44. Saidi, D.; Zaid, B.; Souami, N.; Negache, M.; Si Ahmed, A. Microstructure and fracture mode of a martensitic stainless steel steam turbine blade characterized via scanning auger microscopy and potentiodynamic polarization. In Proceedings of the International Symposium on Advanced Materials (ISAM 2013), Islamabad, Pakistan, 23–27 September 2013; pp. 1–9.

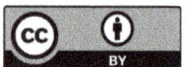

© 2020 by the authors. Licensee MDPI, Basel, Switzerland. This article is an open access article distributed under the terms and conditions of the Creative Commons Attribution (CC BY) license (http://creativecommons.org/licenses/by/4.0/).

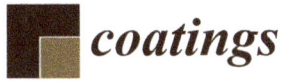

Article

Repetitive Impact Wear Behaviors of the Tempered 25Cr3Mo2NiWV Fe-Based Steel

Cheng Zhang [1,†], Pu Li [1,†], Hui Dong [2,*], Dongliang Jin [1,*], Jinfeng Huang [3], Feng Mao [1] and Chong Chen [1]

1. National Joint Engineering Research Center for Abrasion Control and Molding of Metal Materials, School of Materials Science and Engineering, Henan University of Science and Technology, Luoyang 471003, China; zhangch06@126.com (C.Z.); lp771597120@163.com (P.L.); maofeng718@163.com (F.M.); chenchong8812@163.com (C.C.)
2. School of Materials Science and Engineering, Xi'an Shiyou University, Xi'an 710065, China
3. State Key Laboratory for Advanced Metals and Materials, University of Science and Technology Beijing, Beijing 100083, China; ustbhuangjf@163.com
* Correspondence: donghui@xsyu.edu.cn (H.D.); ziranheping@163.com (D.J.); Tel.: +86-29-8838-2607 (H.D.); +86-731-6427-0020 (D.J.)
† These authors contributed equally to this work.

Received: 9 December 2019; Accepted: 23 January 2020; Published: 26 January 2020

Abstract: This study aimed to reveal the impact wear behaviors of tempered 25Cr3Mo2NiWV steel. The specimens were subject to various heat treatment processes for generating different mechanical and wear properties. The impact wear tests were performed with an MLD-10 dynamic abrasive wear tester. Worn surface morphologies and micro-cracks of the cross-sections were analyzed by optical microscope and scanning electron microscope. The Vickers hardness of the sample and the impact wear mechanism were also analyzed. The steel with the best combination of hardness and toughness had the lowest wear. With the increase of wear time, the dominant wear mechanism varied from slight plastic deformation to micro-cutting and adhesive wear. Finally, micro fatigue peeling occurred. After impact wear, the cracks could initiate from the surface or the sub-surface. Micrographs of the crack in the cross-section demonstrated two different propagation modes of fatigue fractures. The results showed that the strength and toughness of steel affected the crack propagation, surface spalling, and wear failure mechanism during impact wear.

Keywords: impact wear; steel; hardness; toughness; micro fatigue; cracks

1. Introduction

Die steel possesses proper hardness and toughness, good tempering resistance, and moderate cost; thus, it is widely utilized in the manufacturing industry [1]. Wear is one of the main causes of mechanical parts failure [2–6]. In working processes, cyclic mechanical loadings are applied to dies, finally leading to serious damage to the workpiece. The impact wear can alter the dimensional accuracy of the mold, and reduce the surface quality of machine parts, failing the production requirements. Moreover, the impact wear can cause mold fracture and shorten its service life. Therefore, the behavior of impact wear has become one of the important concerns for steel researchers [7–9].

Generally, the wear behavior of given steel has a close relationship with its heat-treatment process, hardness, and toughness [10]. Therefore, the researches on the effect of heat-treatment on the wear behavior are of importance to engineering. Heat treatment can change the mechanical properties of the steel and thus enhance their wear resistance [10–14]. To study the characteristics and the law of the impact wear failure of the test steel, it is tempered at different temperatures to produce various combinations of hardness and toughness.

The wear test is carried out for alloys with an dynamic abrasive wear tester (MLD-10, Zhangjiakou, China). In this test, the circular friction pair rotates under the testing machine. The specimen is fixed on the top, reciprocating up and down, and the repeated impact wear process is carried out within a set time.

Due to good hardenability and fatigue properties, the secondary hardening steel has been widely employed in mold manufacturing [1,15,16]. As an exploratory work [17], the previous research studied the effects of tempering temperature on mechanical properties, total weight loss, and surface morphology of one kind of secondary hardening steel. To obtain better comprehensive properties, the 25Cr3Mo2NiWV steel was developed through the adjustment of elements. On the basis of improved steel, the wear behaviors in different time stages, including weight loss, surface wear morphology, and wear mechanism, were studied more carefully. Besides, different types of cracks were found on the surface and sub-surface of the specimen. In this paper, the impact wear process in different periods was studied more deeply, which was more significant to understand the impact wear behavior of this kind of steel.

2. Experiment

2.1. Material and Heat Treatment

The chemical composition of the 25Cr3Mo2NiWV steel was 0.23 wt.% C, 0.06 wt.% Si, 2.97 wt.% Cr, 2.35 wt.% Mo, 1.05 wt.% Ni, 0.39 wt.% W, 0.27 wt.% V, and remainder Fe. The steel was prepared by vacuum melting combined with the electro-slag remelting process and forged by 400 kg air hammer into Φ70 mm bar stocks. The stable structure of the steel was obtained after annealing at 870 °C for 2 h. The austenitizing and tempering heat treatment conditions and mechanical properties of the steel are listed in Table 1. Due to the secondary hardening effect, the hardness of 25Cr3Mo2NiWV steel increased slightly when tempered at 550 °C [18].

The hardness of the tempered steel was obtained using a Rockwell hardness tester (HR150A, Shandong, China) with an applied load of 150 kg, and the applied load was 200 g for a Vickers hardness tester (HVS-1000A, Shandong, China). The impact toughness test was conducted on an impact test machine (JBDW-300D, Qingdao, China), and the impact specimen was a u-shaped notched sample with a size of 10 mm × 10 mm × 55 mm. All of the mechanical properties were averaged from three results with standard error within ±5% variation.

Table 1. Heat treatment conditions and mechanical properties of the steel.

No.	Condition	Rockwell Hardness (HRC)	Impact Toughness (J·mm^{-2})
1	T1: austenitized at 980 °C for 1.5 h and quenching in water at room temperature, followed by tempering at 300 °C for 2 h	45.9 ± 0.4	54.5 ± 3.7
2	T2: same quenching as T1, tempering at 550 °C for 2 h	46.7 ± 0.5	69.8 ± 3.2
3	T3: same quenching as T1, tempering at 680 °C for 2 h	32.3 ± 0.7	102.6 ± 3.4

2.2. Impact Wear Test

An MLD-10 impact tester was used to investigate the effect of mechanical properties on the impact wear resistance of the 25Cr3Mo2NiWV steel, as shown in Figure 1. The 10 kg impact hammer falling with a height of 4 mm corresponding to impact energy of 4 J was used for the tests without abrasive particles and lubricants. Impact frequencies and rotation frequencies were 200 times/min and 200 r/min, respectively. The upper specimen with the size of 10 mm × 10 mm × 30 mm was cut from the tempered bars, and the lower specimen was a quenched GCr15 steel with a size of Φ50 mm (hardness of 60 HRC).

The chemical composition of the GCr15 steel was 1.02 wt.% C, 1.59 wt.% Cr, 0.33 wt.% Si, 0.30 wt.% Mn, and remainder Fe.

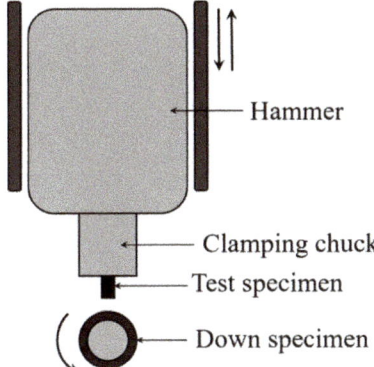

Figure 1. Schematic illustration of the MLD-10 impact wear tester.

Before wear tests, the specimen was ground by 600 grit silicon carbide paper, and then cleaned ultrasonically in the alcohol for 20 min. During the wear test, the specimens were weighed every 15 min using an electronic balance with an accuracy of 0.00001 g. The wear mass loss was average from three results for each period.

2.3. Microscopic Analysis

The morphologies and chemical composition of the worn surface were analyzed via a scanning electron microscope (SEM, TESCAN-VEGA3SBH, Warrendale, PA, USA) and the energy spectrometer (EDS). The cross-section of the worn surface was ground using a final 2000 grit silicon carbide paper and then corroded with 8% nitric acid alcohol. The cracks in the cross-section were studied using optical microscopy (OM, OLYMPUS-BX51M, Tokyo, Japan) and SEM. The micro-hardness was tested three times on the cross-section by Vickers hardness tester (HVS-1000A, Shandong, China).

3. Results and Discussion

3.1. Wear Loss of 25Cr3Mo2NiWV Steel with Time

Figure 2 shows the wear loss as a function of time for the steel tempered at different temperatures. The weight loss increased with time for all of the specimens. The weight losses of these three types of specimens increased slowly in the first 15 min. However, the increment of the wear loss increased rapidly after 15 min, which was caused by the rough surface from the microstructural aspect [19]. The real contact area was small between the upper and lower specimens during the initial stage of friction, only some undulations on the surface contacted with each other. With the proceeding of impact wear, the protrusions would undergo plastic deformation and adhesive tear under the impact force and shear stress when the stress is greater than the yield strength of the material [19,20]. The protrusions could partially break away from the wear system and result in weight loss, and the debris would form hard particles to cause micro-cutting.

The hardness of the tempered steel at 300 and 550 °C was higher than that tempered at 680 °C, resulting in a lower weight loss caused by micro-cutting during a long-time test. Due to higher hardness, the embedding of the hard particles that broke away from the steel surface was difficult, and its embedding depth was small under the impact force. Furthermore, the particles with shallow embedding depth that formed cutting effect could not slide long-distance on the steel surface, owing to the instantaneity of the impact load [21]. At the initial stage of the wear test for the steel tempered at 680 °C, the particles were easy to be embedded into the matrix and plowed the steel surface by tangential friction [22]. However, the plowed metal could be rapidly pressed back into the steel matrix, resulting from the high plasticity and toughness of the matrix. Therefore, its wear loss was also low at the initial wear stage.

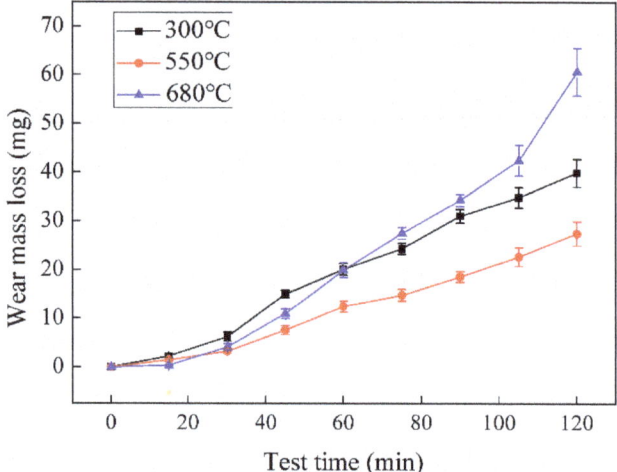

Figure 2. Weight loss as a function of wear time for the specimens tempered at different temperatures.

As the wear time increased, the ability of plastic deformation decreased for the steel surface, and the damage on the worn surface accumulated under the repeated impact. Cracks were generated by the large stress concentration in the grain boundary of the matrix, which could propagate and connect to form peeling during the test [23]. This might be the reason that the wear rate of the steels was higher after 15 min, as shown in Figure 2.

3.2. Evolution of the Worn Surface Morphology

According to the results from Figure 2, the analysis of the wear mechanism was mainly focused on the steel tempered at 680 °C due to its highest wear loss. Figure 3 shows the surface morphologies of the steel tempered at 680 °C with different wear times. The worn surface was relatively flat after the impact test for 5 min. The slight impact indentation was uniformly distributed on the surface, and some adhesive marks are presented in Figure 3a. The surface appeared obvious plastic deformation after a 10-min test, as shown in Figure 3b. The small protrusions could act as hard abrasive particles at the early stage of wear and scratch the surface under the impact load, resulting in some grooves with adhesive tear marks [24,25]. The wear mechanisms were mainly micro-cutting. With the increasing time, serious plastic deformation appeared on the surface, the widths and the depths of the grooves were expanded, leading to an increase of the wear loss. At the same time, the material in the groove could be pushed onto both sides of the groove to form a plastic ridge [26,27]. Besides, the scale-shaped morphology could be seen because of severe adhesive wear [28], and sheet-shaped debris with a size of ~15 μm could be observed locally, as shown in Figure 3c.

Figure 4 shows the surface morphology and EDS analysis of 25Cr3Mo2NiWV steel after tempering at 680 °C and wear test for 15 min. The contents of C and Si elements in the grinding material (GCr15) were higher than those of 25Cr3Mo2NiWV steel. During the adhesive wear, a part of the asperities on the surface of grinding material was torn and transferred to the worn surface of the impact specimen. In Figure 4, the content of C and Si elements in the adhesive wear area was higher, proving the adhesive features. Besides, the impact wear could rise the local temperature of the sample surface, leading to oxidation. The oxygen content in the adhesion region was higher, which was consistent with the results of So [29].

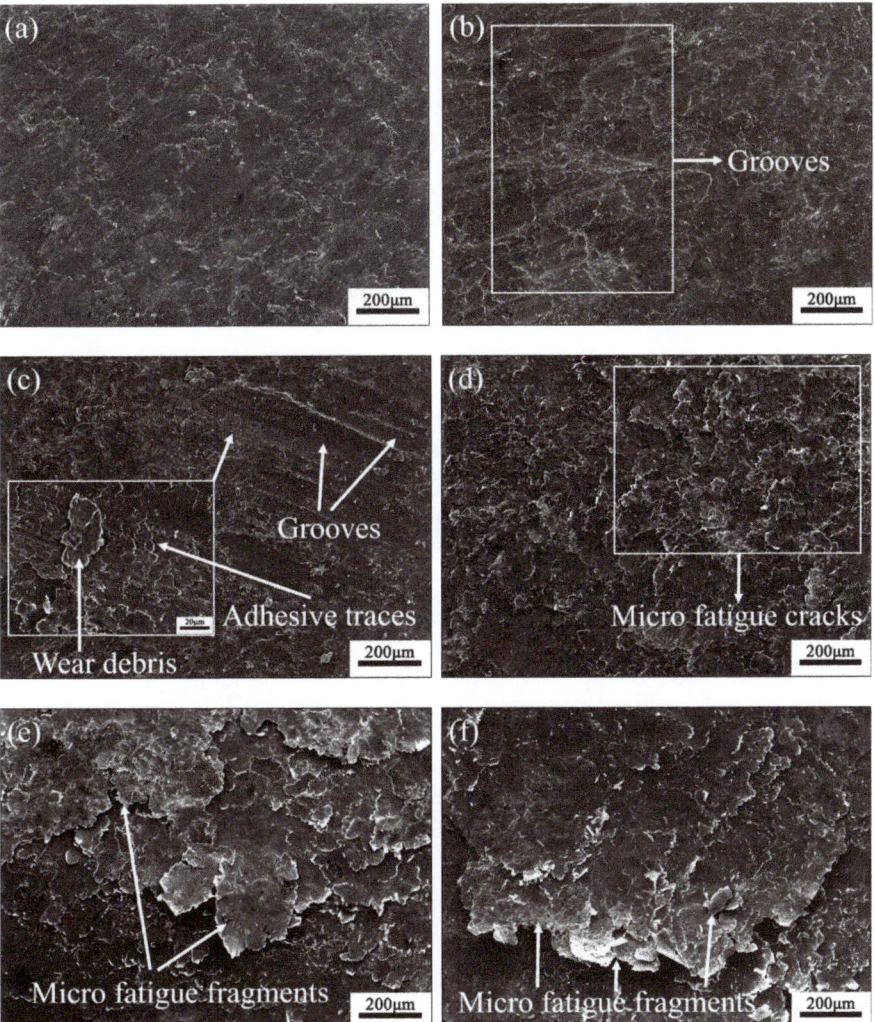

Figure 3. Surface morphologies of the steel tempered at 680 °C for different impact wear times, (**a**) 5 min; (**b**) 10 min; (**c**) 15 min; (**d**) 30 min; (**e**) 60 min; (**f**) 120 min.

At 30 min, no signs of adhesive wear were presented on the steel surface, while after frequent dynamic impact on the sample surface, a large number of micro fatigue cracks were observed, as shown in Figure 3d. There were mainly two reasons for the formation of the micro fatigue cracks. Firstly, the micro friction traces after adhesive wear become micro-cracks under the impact force and then propagate to form micro fatigue cracks [30]. Secondly, the deformation degree of the plastic ridge on both sides of the groove increases and transforms into an extrusion hardening ridge under repeated impact. The root of the hardened edge is prone to crack due to strain fatigue [31].

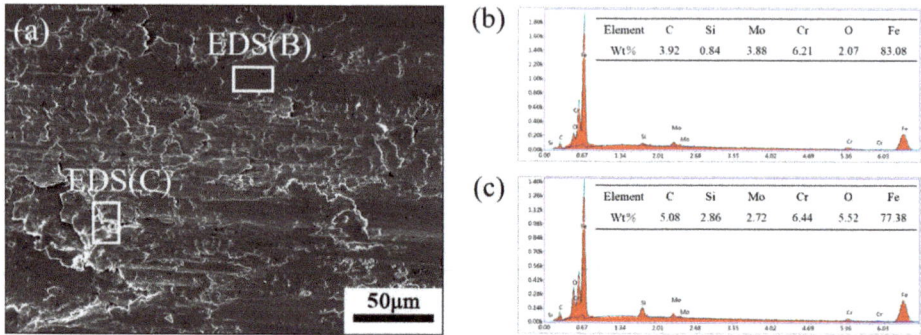

Figure 4. Surface wear morphology and EDS analysis of 680 °C tempered samples after 15 min wear. (**a**) Micro morphology of worn surface; (**b**) EDS analysis of region marked with EDS(B); (**c**) EDS analysis of region marked with EDS(C).

For the 60-min wear test, the worn surface was hardened under the impact, and the fatigue crack was easier to develop. It could be seen that small cracks propagated and coalesced to form large cracks, and the lip at the front of the fragment had the potential to peel off under the shear stress, as shown by the arrow in Figure 3e. At the 120-min test, the surface morphology was quite rough, filled with fish-scale fragments, as shown in Figure 3f. There were fractures between the fatigue fragments, and the wear mechanism was mainly micro fatigue peeling wear.

Besides, based on the morphologies in Figure 3, it also could be deduced that the hardness and the toughness of the 25Cr3Mo2NiWV steel both dramatically affected its impact wear resistance. Due to high hardness, the depth and width of the groove were small, and the weight loss by micro-cutting was correspondingly low. With high toughness, the fatigue crack was not easily formed, resulting in the fatigue peeling under the impact wear [32]. Therefore, the high hardness and toughness were beneficial to promote the wear resistance of the steel.

During the wear test of the 25Cr3Mo2NiWV steel, the dominant wear mechanisms varied from the slight plastic deformation to micro-cutting and adhesive wear, finally to micro fatigue peeling wear in the dynamic impact wear. Due to the different hardness and toughness, the main wear mechanism varied with the different specimen surface in the same wear time, leading to different wear weight losses.

3.3. Effects of Tempering Temperature on the Worn Surface Morphologies

Figure 5 displays the worn surface morphologies of the steels with different tempering temperatures after wear for a different time. The typical fish-scale fragments were observed on all surfaces. The surface was the flattest for the specimen tempered at 550 °C with the wear time of 60 min, and no fatigue peeling presents in Figure 5(b1). The worn surfaces of the steels tempered at 300 and 680 °C were quite rough, and the size of the fragments was large, as shown in Figure 5(a1,c1). The fish scale fractures along the direction of shear stress and the secondary micro-cracks could be observed, which indicated that a large part of fish scales had peeled off, resulting in weight loss and poor wear resistance.

For 120 min wear time, the surface morphologies of all specimens were almost the same as those worn for 60 min, but their fatigue peeling was more serious, as shown in Figure 5(a2,c2). Except for the steel tempered at 550 °C, the worn sub-surface layer had been exposed for the other specimens, as marked as 2 in Figure 5 (the area marked as 1 is the initial wear surface). The surface temperature of the specimens could rise owing to impact and friction, decreasing the wear resistance of the surface layer. Besides, due to the low strength and hardness of the steel tempered at 680 °C, its surface morphology was the roughest with the largest peeling off, and the plastic extrusion was found on the cross-section [33], as shown in Figure 6.

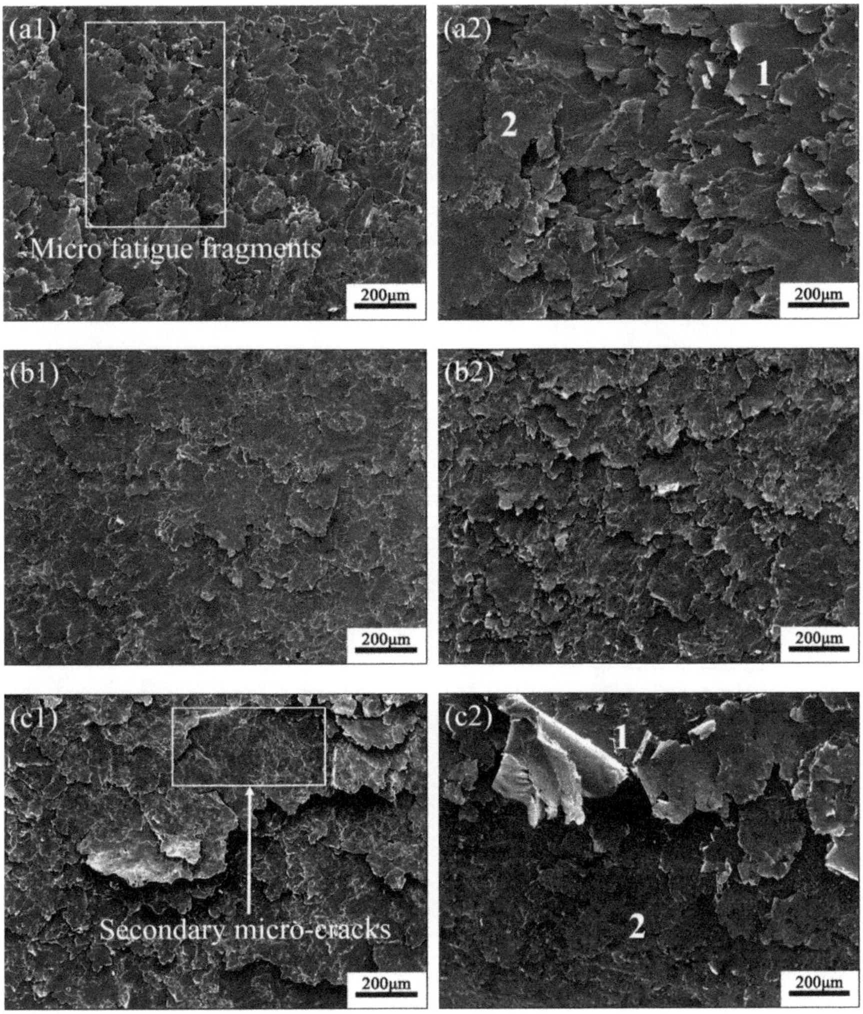

Figure 5. Worn surface morphologies of the tempered steels, (**a1**) 300 °C/60 min and (**a2**) 300 °C/120 min; (**b1**) 550 °C/60 min and (**b2**) 550 °C/120 min; (**c1**) 680 °C/60 min and (**c2**) 680 °C/120 min.

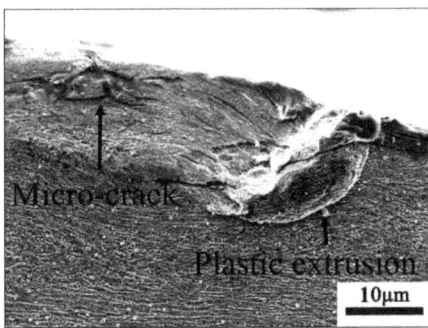

Figure 6. Cross-section morphology of the steel tempered at 680 °C after impact wear for 120 min.

3.4. Mechanism of Crack Initiation and Surface Spalling

Essentially, wear is the process of hardening and peeling off in the worn surface, that is, the process of forming, expanding, and converging of micro-cracks in the surface layer [34]. Table 2 shows the micro-hardness of the cross-sections of the steels tempered at different temperatures. The surface layer experiences serious plastic deformation after impact wear; thus, its hardness is higher than that of the metal matrix.

Table 2. Micro-hardness of surface layer and matrix after wear tests.

Condition	None Heat Treatment	Tempering Temperature (°C)		
		300	550	680
Matrix hardness (HV)	151.0 ± 3.1	439.3 ± 5.5	458.0 ± 6.0	292.3 ± 7.6
Surface hardness (HV)	–	589.0 ± 5.3	572.0 ± 6.2	418.0 ± 9.6
Hardness difference (HV)	–	149.7 ± 2.1	114.0 ± 1.7	125.7 ± 2.5

Figure 7 presents the micrographs of the crack in the cross-section, demonstrating two different propagation modes of the fatigue fractures.

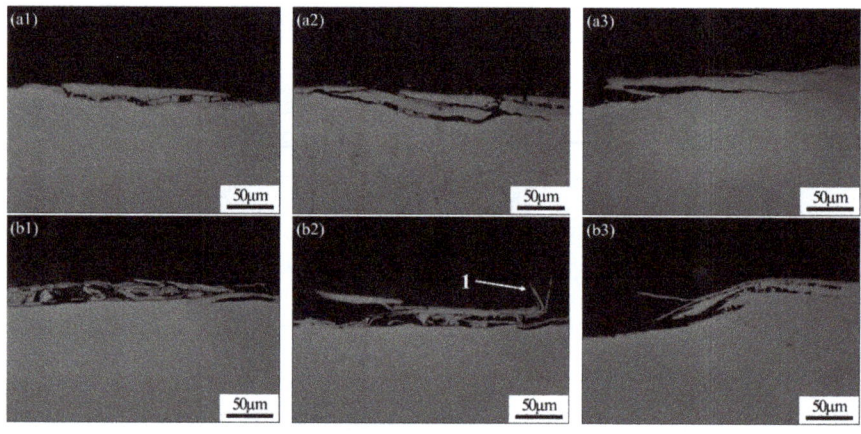

Figure 7. Cross-sectional micrographs of the steels after wear for 120 min. (**a1–a3**) Steel tempered at 300 °C, brittle fatigue fractures; (**b1–b3**) steel tempered at 680 °C, ductile fatigue fractures.

Cracks initiated on the worn surface under impact load (Figure 7(a1,b1)) and then expanded and converged at a small angle into the matrix, finally returning to the surface to cause flake spalling in Figure 7(a2,b2), exposing the sub-surface layer. The cracks in the steel tempered at 300 °C were straight with clear edges in Figure 7(a1,a3), showing a brittle fracture due to high hardness and low toughness. Combined with work hardening, the surface became harder and more brittle, obstructing the stress release and aggravating the expansion of fatigue cracks. The difference of the micro-hardness between the surface and matrix for the steel tempered at 300 °C was the largest, 149.7 HV, indicating poor coordination between the surface and the matrix. Once the fatigue crack initiated, it would expand rapidly along with the surface layer under the shear stress, ultimately causing the surface layer to peel off.

The cross-section of the worn steel tempered at 680 °C is shown in Figure 7(b1,b3). The higher tempering temperature induced a higher toughness, and the resistance to crack propagation was enhanced. Consequently, the cracks were short and curved, showing a plastic fracture mode. However, the higher tempering temperature decreased the strength of the metal matrix, leading to low resistance to plastic deformation. The micro-cracks were more easily to initiate from the grooves under impact load [35]. Besides, the fatigue scaling marked by arrow 1 in Figure 7(b2) did not break away during impact wear, also indicating a plastic fracture mechanism. The plastic scale could be folded before peeling off, as shown in Figure 5(c2).

After the test, the surface cracks and spalling of the specimen tempered at 550 °C were less, as shown in Figure 5(b1,b2). The crack initiation and propagation were evident.

Figure 8 shows the different micro-cracks in the cross-sections of the steels tempered at 550 °C after impact wear for a different time. Under the normal and shear stress, severe plastic deformation developed in the surface layer, forming the typical streamline under high strain [36].

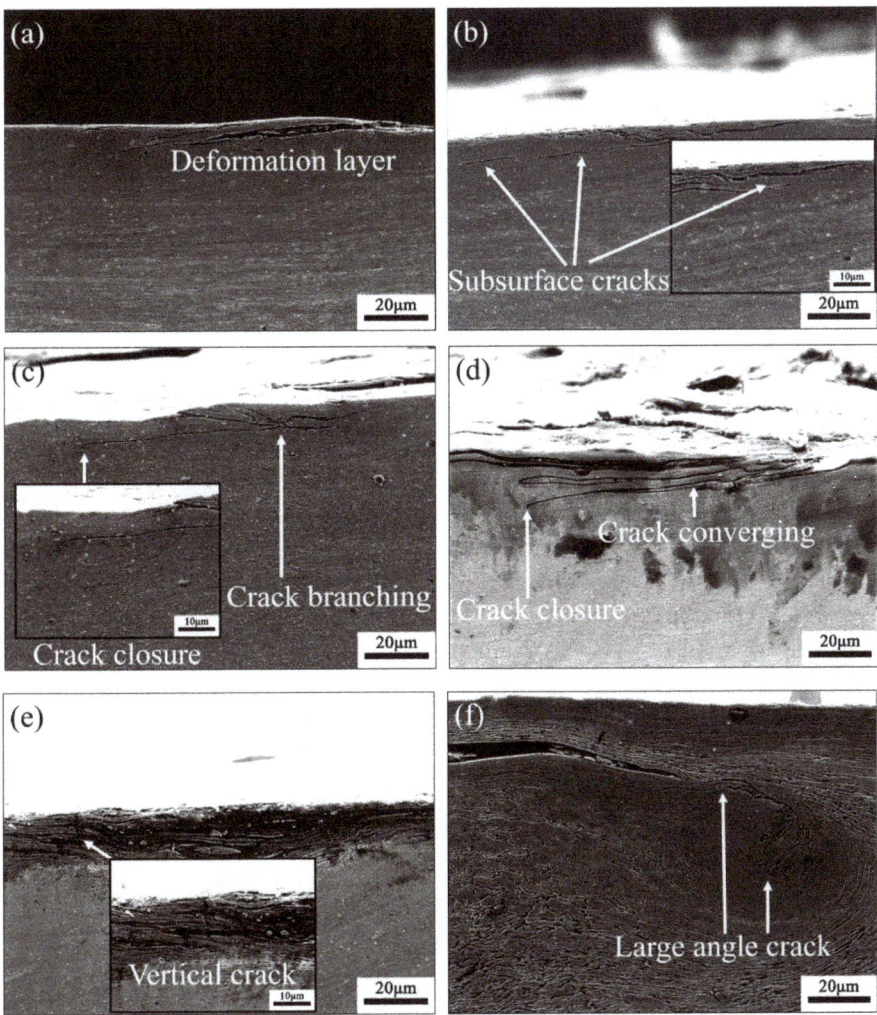

Figure 8. Micro-cracks in the cross-sections of the steels tempered at 550 °C after wear for different time, (**a**) 30 min, crack expanding inward; (**b**) 30 min, sub-surface crack expanding outwards; (**c**) 60 min, crack propagating; (**d**) 60 min, crack converging; (**e**) 120 min, vertical crack; (**f**) 120 min, sub-surface large-angle crack.

Cracks in the dense streamline could expand inward (Figure 8a) and outward (Figure 8b) and produce branches (Figure 8c), even converge to form a long curved crack (Figure 8d). These kinds of cracks were mainly initiated along with the interface of martensitic. The cracks near the surface almost expanded parallel to the surface.

From Figure 8b,d, it could be found that the expansion of the cracks near the surface paused after branching in the metal matrix. Moreover, the cracks near the surface could be closed by large compressive stress [37]. Figure 8e shows a vertical crack without branching in the surface layer. The vertical cracks often converged with the crack parallel to the surface. Figure 8f presents a large angle crack formed in the sub-surface. According to the fatigue theory [38], when the metal material is impacted, the micro defects, such as dislocations, first form in the sub-surface under the impact, and then evolve into cracks, finally resulting in spalling. However, the lath of the martensite has a high density of dislocations, which could form a large number of dislocation tangles and dislocation walls during impact wear [39,40], leading to the development of the large angle crack, as shown in Figure 8f.

4. Conclusions

Both hardness and toughness could affect the wear properties of steel. Hardness has a greater influence on wear properties. The steel with the best combination of hardness and toughness has the lowest wear weight loss.

With the increase of wear time, the dominant wear mechanisms of all tempered steels vary from the slight plastic deformation to micro-cutting and adhesive wear, finally to micro fatigue peeling wear. Due to the different hardness and toughness, the main wear mechanism of three tempered specimens are different during the same wear time, resulting in different wear weight losses.

During impact wear, the fatigue cracks could initiate from the surface and the sub-surface, and then propagate and converge to form fatigue delamination. The fatigue cracks in the cross-section show the characteristics of the toughness and brittleness. The brittle fatigue fractures mainly appear in the steels with high hardness. However, the ductile fatigue fractures mainly occur in the steels with high toughness. With a good combination of strength and toughness, the surface cracks and spalling of the specimen are the least.

Author Contributions: Conceptualization and investigation, C.Z.; data curation and investigation, P.L.; writing—review and editing, H.D.; writing—original draft, D.J.; formal analysis, J.H.; data curation, F.M.; investigation, C.C. All authors have read and agreed to the published version of the manuscript.

Funding: The work was supported by the National Key R&D Program of China (No. 2016YFB0300701), Key Scientific and Technological Project of Henan Province (Nos. 182102210043 and 192102210009).

Conflicts of Interest: The authors declare no conflict of interest.

References

1. Zhu, Z.Y. Property data collection of common hot working die steels used in China. *Mater. Mech. Eng.* **2001**, *26*, 42–46.
2. Koiprasert, H.; Dumrongrattana, S.; Niranatlumpong, P. Thermally sprayed coatings for protection of fretting wear. *Wear* **2004**, *257*, 1–7. [CrossRef]
3. Jiang, Z.; Mao, Z.; Zhang, Y.; Zhang, J. A study on dynamic response and diagnosis method of the wear on connecting rod bush. *J. Fail. Anal. Prev.* **2017**, *17*, 812–822. [CrossRef]
4. Wei, S.; Xu, L. Review on research progress of steel and iron wear-resistant material. *Acta Metall. Sin.* **2019**. [CrossRef]
5. Luong, L.H.S.; Heijkoop, T. The influence of scale on friction in hot metal working. *Wear* **1981**, *71*, 93–102. [CrossRef]
6. Barrau, O.; Boher, C.; Gras, R.; Rezai-Aria, F. Analysis of the friction and wear behavior of hot work tool steel for forging. *Wear* **2003**, *255*, 1444–1454. [CrossRef]
7. Liu, Y.; Janssen, G.C.A.M. Impact wear of structural steel with yield strength of 235 MPa in various liquids. *Coatings* **2017**, *7*, 237. [CrossRef]
8. Yilmaz, H.; Sadeler, R. Impact wear behavior of ball burnished 316L stainless steel. *Surf. Coat. Technol.* **2019**, *363*, 369–378. [CrossRef]

9. Wang, Z.; Cai, Z.; Sun, Y.; Peng, J.; Zhu, M. Low velocity impact wear behavior of MoS2/Pb nanocomposite coating under controlled kinetic energy. *Surf. Coat. Technol.* **2017**, *326*, 53–62. [CrossRef]
10. Cui, X.H.; Wang, S.Q.; Wei, M.X.; Yang, Z.R. Wear characteristics and mechanisms of H13 steel with various tempered structures. *J. Mater. Eng. Perform.* **2011**, *20*, 1055–1062. [CrossRef]
11. Xu, L.; Wei, S.; Xiao, F.; Zhou, H.; Zhang, G.; Li, J. Effects of carbides on abrasive wear properties and failure behaviors of high speed steels with different alloy element content. *Wear* **2017**, *376–377*, 968–974. [CrossRef]
12. Xu, L.; Xiao, F.; Wei, S.; Liu, D.; Zhou, H.; Zhang, G.; Zhou, Y. Microstructure and wear properties of high-speed steel with high molybdenum content under rolling-sliding wear. *Tribol. Int.* **2017**, *116*, 39–46. [CrossRef]
13. Xu, L.; Wei, S.; Xing, J.; Long, R. Effects of carbon content and sliding ratio on wear behavior of high-vanadium high-speed steel (HVHSS) under high-stress rolling sliding contact. *Tribol. Int.* **2014**, *70*, 34–41. [CrossRef]
14. Xu, L.; Wei, S.; Han, M.; Long, R. Effect of carbides on wear characterization of high-alloy steels under high-stress rolling-sliding condition. *Tribol. Trans.* **2014**, *57*, 631–636. [CrossRef]
15. Hao, X.; Pan, M.L; Liu, X.F. Effect of cerium on microstructure and wearing resistance of 5CrMnMo hot working die steel. *Adv. Mater. Res.* **2011**, *284–286*, 1615–1620. [CrossRef]
16. Kuang, J.X.; Wang, X.H.; Liu, A.M.; Zhu, H.S. Study on the complex strengthening processes of 5Cr2NiMoVSi steel large hot forging dies. *Adv. Mater. Res.* **2011**, *189–193*, 1056–1061. [CrossRef]
17. Zhang, C.; Li, P.; Wei, S.; You, L.; Wang, X.; Mao, F.; Jin, D.; Chen, C.; Pan, K.; Luo, C.; et al. Effect of tempering temperature on impact wear behavior of 30Cr3Mo2WNi hot-working die steel. *Front. Mater.* **2019**, *6*, 149. [CrossRef]
18. Chen, X.F.; Yao, Z.H.; Huang, J.F.; Zhang, J.; Dong, J.X. Thermodynamic calculation of precipitated phase in 25Cr3Mo2NiWVNb steel. *China Sciencepaper* **2017**, *12*, 1178–1183.
19. Jahanmir, S.; Suh, N.P.; Abrahamson, E.P., II. Abrahamson. The delamination theory of wear and the wear of a composite surface. *Wear* **1975**, *32*, 33–49. [CrossRef]
20. Wei, M.; Wang, S.; Wang, L.; Chen, K. Effect of microstructures on elevated-temperature wear resistance of a hot working die steel. *J. Iron Steel Res. Int.* **2001**, *18*, 47–53. [CrossRef]
21. Bialobrzeska, B.; Kostencki, P. Abrasive wear characteristics of selected low-alloy boron steels as measured in both field experiments and laboratory tests. *Wear* **2015**, *328–329*, 149–159. [CrossRef]
22. Wang, X.; Chen, Y.; Wei, S.; Zuo, L.; Mao, F. Effect of carbon content on abrasive impact wear behavior of Cr-Si-Mn low alloy wear resistant cast steels. *Front. Mater.* **2019**, *6*, 153. [CrossRef]
23. Laird, G., II; Collins, W.K.; Blickensderfer, R. Crack propagation and spalling of white cast iron balls subjected to repeated impacts. *Wear* **1988**, *124*, 217–235. [CrossRef]
24. Archard, J.F.; Hirst, W. The wear of metals under unlubricated conditions. *Proc. Math. Phys. Eng. Sci.* **1956**, *236*, 397–410.
25. Xu, J. Study on the coated tool disability and the work-piece surface quality in high speed cutting. *Key Eng. Mater.* **2010**, *431–432*, 397–400. [CrossRef]
26. Liu, C.-H.; Sun, G.-D.; Xiong, L.; Yang, X.-Q. Effect of heat treatment process on impact wear property and mechanism of SKD11 steel. *J. Iron Steel Res.* **2018**, *30*, 199–205.
27. Ding, H.; Cui, F.; Du, X. Effect of component and microstructure on impact wear property and mechanism of steels in corrosive condition. *Mater. Sci. Eng. A* **2006**, *421*, 161–167. [CrossRef]
28. Wei, M.X.; Wang, S.Q.; Wang, L.; Cui, X.H.; Chen, K.M. Effect of tempering conditions on wear resistance in various wear mechanisms of H13 steel. *Tribol. Int.* **2011**, *44*, 898–905. [CrossRef]
29. So, H.; Yu, D.S.; Chuang, C.Y. Formation and wear mechanism of tribo-oxides and the regime of oxidational wear of steel. *Wear* **2002**, *253*, 1004–1015. [CrossRef]
30. Sasada, T.; Oike, M.; Emori, N. The effect of abrasive grain size on the transition between abrasive and adhesive wear. *Wear* **1984**, *97*, 291–302. [CrossRef]
31. Dai, P.Q.; Huang, S.X. Effect of heat treatment on the impact abrasive wear resistance of medium carbon alloy steel. *Heat Treat. Met.* **1998**, *12*, 19–21.
32. Fricke, R.W.; Allen, C. Repetitive impact wear of steels. *Wear* **1993**, *162–164*, 837–847. [CrossRef]
33. So, H.; Chen, H.M.; Chen, L.W. Extrusion wear and transition of wear mechanisms of steel. *Wear* **2008**, *265*, 1142–1148. [CrossRef]
34. Rastegar, V.; Karimi, A. Surface and subsurface deformation of wear-resistant steels exposed to impact wear. *J. Mater. Eng. Perform.* **2014**, *23*, 927–936. [CrossRef]

35. Huang, J.F.; Fang, H.-S.; Xu, P.; Zheng, Y.K. Effect of Si on wear resistance of bainitic cast steel under high stress impact. *J. Iron Steel Res.* **2001**, *13*, 40–45.
36. Alpas, A.T.; Embury, J.D. The role of subsurface deformation and strain localization on the sliding wear behaviour of laminated composites. *Wear* **1991**, *146*, 285–300. [CrossRef]
37. Yang, Y.-Y.; Fang, H.-S.; Zheng, Y.-K; Yang, Z.-G.; Jiang, Z.-L. The failure models induced by white layers during impact wear. *Wear* **1995**, *185*, 17–22. [CrossRef]
38. Suh, N.P. An overview of the delamination theory of wear. *Wear* **1977**, *44*, 1–16. [CrossRef]
39. Peng, S.; Song, R.; Sun, T.; Yang, F.; Deng, P.; Wu, C. Surface failure behavior of 70Mn martensite steel under abrasive impact wear. *Wear* **2016**, *362–363*, 129–134. [CrossRef]
40. Peng, S.; Song, R.; Sun, T.; Pei, Z.; Cai, C.; Feng, Y.; Tan, Z. Wear behavior and hardening mechanism of novel lightweight Fe–25.1Mn–6.6Al–1.3C steel under impact abrasion conditions. *Tribol. Lett.* **2016**, *64*. [CrossRef]

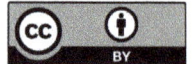

© 2020 by the authors. Licensee MDPI, Basel, Switzerland. This article is an open access article distributed under the terms and conditions of the Creative Commons Attribution (CC BY) license (http://creativecommons.org/licenses/by/4.0/).

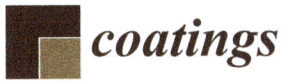

Article

An Erosion-Corrosion Investigation of Coated Steel for Applications in the Oil and Gas Field, Based on Bipolar Electrochemistry

Claudio Mele [1],*, Francesca Lionetto [1],* and Benedetto Bozzini [2]

1 Dipartimento di Ingegneria dell'Innovazione, Università del Salento, via Monteroni, 73100 Lecce, Italy
2 Dipartimento di Energia, Politecnico di Milano, Via Lambruschini 4, 20156 Milano, Italy; benedetto.bozzini@polimi.it
* Correspondence: claudio.mele@unisalento.it (C.M.); francesca.lionetto@unisalento.it (F.L.); Tel.: +39-832-297-269 (C.M.)

Received: 10 December 2019; Accepted: 19 January 2020; Published: 21 January 2020

Abstract: In this research, a simple experimental apparatus based on a bipolar electrode (BPE) configuration was set up, in order to tackle erosion-corrosion problems of materials of interest in the oil and gas field. As a case study, the resistance to erosion and corrosion of carbon steel samples coated by Electroless Nickel Plating and by thermo-sprayed coating with the high velocity oxy fuel (HVOF) process was investigated. The main objective was to demonstrate if this simple, contactless technique could be applied to effectively discriminate the erosion-corrosion behavior of different materials in a vast range of experimental conditions. In fact, by means of polarization curves, visual inspection and morphological analysis by scanning electron microscope (SEM), the effects due to erosion-corrosion by solid particles, by fluid and those due to simple erosion were evaluated.

Keywords: bipolar electrochemistry; erosion-corrosion; oil and gas

---

1. Introduction

The oil and gas production field presents aggressive conditions in terms of erosion and corrosion. Careful attention must be given to the material selection at every stage of the design, construction and operation of piping systems and their accessories, such as bends, elbows, tees and valves [1–5]. It is therefore mandatory that the materials of such components have high erosion and corrosion resistance combined with high mechanical strength.

The erosion-corrosion process depends on the corrosive fluid, on the nature and chemical composition of metal and alloy and on the surface condition. The protective film on the metal surface could be swept away by the rapid movement of the processing fluid, possibly also containing solid particulate. Several preventive methods can be employed: appropriate design of shape or geometry to prevent turbulence, alteration of environment as settling and filtration to remove solid particles or reduction of temperature, use of highly corrosion-resistant materials, rarely cathodic protection and use of appropriate coatings [1–3,6].

The state-of-the-art of the materials used for coating components subject to erosion-corrosion involves the use of various thermal spray coating processes, including HVOF (high velocity oxy fuel), EArc (electric arc spray) and APS (atmospheric plasma spray) [7,8]. The coating applied by thermal-spraying processes have numerous advantages: they act as a barrier between the substrate and the aggressive marine or industrial environment, they are able to protect equipment and structures, they reduce friction between contacting surfaces, they can provide a cosmetic finishing, they can properly modify chemical, mechanical, thermal, electronic and optical properties of materials and their application on low-cost substrates results in increased efficiency and cost savings [7–9]. Another quite common coating technology in the oil and gas industry is related to Electroless Nickel Plating (ENP), used to improve corrosion and wear resistance of components in contact with high aggressiveness fluids. The process, based on immersion of the components into a plating bath, is an autocatalytic method in which Ni^{2+} ions in solution are deposited through the oxidation of a chemical compound or reducing agent, typically, sodium hypophosphite. Being an electroless process (i.e., no need for electrodes and current/potential supply), ENP allows for obtaining full coverage of hidden or low-accessibility surfaces and a very good coating uniformity. Although several studies are available in the literature on the erosion-corrosion performance of coatings, they mainly refer to specific coatings or coating-substrate systems and to particular experimental conditions [7–15].

Erosion-corrosion processes involve complex mechanical and electrochemical mechanisms whose combined action often results in a significant increase in material degradation [1,16–18]. The degradation mechanism is affected by factors controlling both corrosion and erosion. Their interaction may result in a synergistic behavior, where erosion may enhance the corrosion rate, or in an antagonistic behavior, where oxidation can slow down the erosion rate [1,14,19,20]. In the classical approach, the synergism is defined as the difference between the total corrosion-wear mass loss and the sum of the corrosion and wear mass losses, measured separately [18]. The interaction between erosion and corrosion has been investigated using various electrochemical and non-electrochemical methods. Non-electrochemical sensors based on the electrical resistance technique and acoustic sense technique have been developed to probe the erosion-corrosion behavior, though they have limitations in providing detailed information of the erosion and corrosion processes and their synergistic effects [21]. Electrochemical measurements, such as potentiodynamic polarization, open circuit potential measurements, ellipsometry, electrochemical impedance spectroscopy and electrochemical noise methods, give significant information about erosion-corrosion mechanisms, which greatly affect the electrochemical state of the surfaces [18]. Electrochemical techniques enable us to determine the effect of wear on the active/passive behavior of materials at different potentials and evaluate changes in the kinetics which controls the rate of corrosion [18]. Electrochemical devices based on rotating disc or cylinder electrode and slurry jet impingement facility are frequently used [7–15]. All these test methods are performed with electrochemical cell configurations based on a direct electric contact of the samples with cable connections. However, in the oil and gas industry, the electric contact is often very difficult to apply during the online inspection where it is quite hard to simultaneously control a very large array of electrodes, which sometimes are mobile in solution. To overcome the problem of electric contact, when direct wiring of the sample is not possible and a conventional electrochemical set-up cannot be used, an electrochemical and contactless technique, called bipolar electrochemistry, seems to be appealing for monitoring erosion-corrosion.

Bipolar electrochemistry is a very versatile technique, characterized by the occurrence of concomitant reduction and oxidation processes at the opposite extremities (poles) of an electrode made of electrically conductive material, called a bipolar electrode (BPE), under the application of an external electric field, without a direct ohmic contact [22–24]. In fact, when sufficient voltage is applied to the "driving electrodes", a uniform electric field is present through the electrolytic solution in which a BPE is immersed, and oxidation and reduction reactions occur at the poles of BPE [22,23]. In general, a BPE refers to any conducting object exhibiting oxidation and reduction reactions at the same time. Unlike a classic electrochemical cell with a three-electrode setup, where the driving force of the redox reactions is directly controlled by tuning the potential of the working electrode that is connected to a power supply, in the open bipolar configuration, the conductive substrate is suspended in an electrolytic solution between two feeder electrodes, without any direct physical connection between the substrate and the power supply. By carefully selecting the experimental parameters, electrochemical reactions at the surface of a conducting object can be accurately controlled [22–24]. Recent applications of bipolar electrochemistry focus on sensing, electrografting, electrodissolution, electrodeposition in fields covering chemistry, biology, materials science and device fabrication [24–28].

The aim of this work is to demonstrate the possibility of studying the erosion-corrosion resistance of coatings with a technique—based on the bipolar electrode configuration—that allows us to perform electrochemical measurements without the need of contacting the sample with cable connections, thus imparting notable flexibility to the choice of testing geometries, ambient and conditions. This is a quite novel application of a bipolar electrochemistry technique. In the literature, in fact, a few works report applications to corrosion screening of stainless steel in acidic solutions [29,30], but to the authors' knowledge, the present paper describes the first investigation in the realm of erosion-corrosion.

In this work, a bipolar electrochemistry rig has been set-up to evaluate the resistance to erosion-corrosion of three types of samples: uncoated carbon steel, chosen as the reference material and the same steel, coated with two different methods: ENP (Electroless Nickel Plating) and the thermo-sprayed HVOF process. With the designed experimental set-up, the measurements carried out in aqueous solution containing chlorides and glass microspheres allowed us to distinguish among the effects due to erosion-corrosion by solid particles, those due to erosion-corrosion by fluid and those due to simple erosion.

2. Materials and Methods

To perform the erosion-corrosion studies, electrochemical measurements were carried out by means of an experimental set-up based on a bipolar electrode configuration (Figure 1). The investigated specimens, with 50 × 20 × 10 mm dimensions, were made of carbon steel coated with high phosphorus Electroless Nickel, indicated as ENP, and with a thermo-sprayed coating, consisting of a nickel-base hard alloy with chromium boride dispersion, obtained with the HVOF technique, indicated as Colmonoy 6. In Table 1 chemical composition, thickness, surface roughness and microhardness of the two coatings are reported.

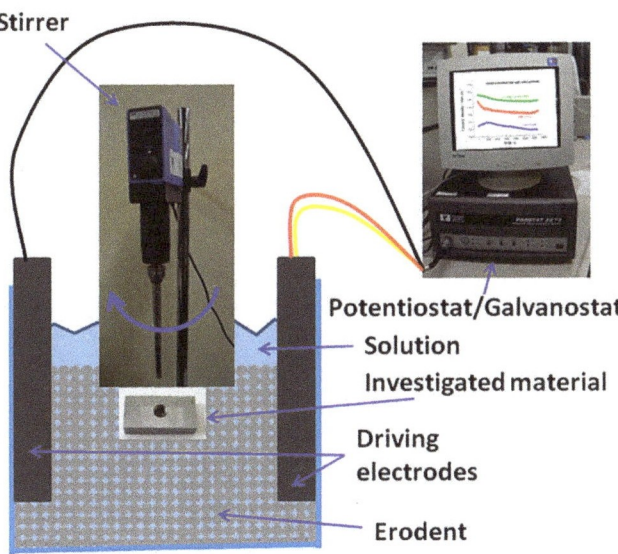

Figure 1. Layout of the experimental rig based on a bipolar electrode configuration, employed to perform erosion-corrosion measurements.

Table 1. Properties of the investigated coatings.

Coating	Chemical Composition	Thickness (μm)	Roughness Ra (μm)	Hardness (HV$_{0.05}$)
ENP [1]	ENP 11%P	80 μm	10 ± 0.6	631 ± 27
Colmonoy 6 [2]	baNi-Cr20-Si5.6-Fe5.7-B2.1-C1.1	350 μm	0.25 ± 0.09	1386 ± 179

[1] ENP: high phosphorus Electroless Nickel coating; [2] Colmonoy 6: thermo-sprayed coating obtained by nigh velocity oxy fuel technique.

The surface roughness was evaluated on 4 profiles with a length of 10 mm and microhardness on a Vickers scale with an applied load of 50 g. The roughness of the ENP-coated sample was higher than Colomonoy6, whereas the hardness of on thermal sprayed coatings was more than double with respect to nickel-plated samples.

As a reference material, samples of uncoated carbon steel were also examined. These prismatic specimens were fabricated with a threaded hole on the back face (see Figure 1), through which they were screwed onto the shaft of an IKA RW20 mechanical stirrer. Two platinized titanium expanded mesh electrodes, exhibiting an area of about 10 cm^2, were used as driving electrodes and fixed to the cell using a rugged Teflon holder, ensuring exact and reproducible positioning. Before measurement, each specimen was mechanically polished with emery papers of different grades down to 1200 grit, degreased with acetone and rinsed with ultrapure water. A test solution containing 600 ppm of Cl$^-$ at room temperature and pH 6 was employed: these relatively mild conditions were selected in order not to over-emphasize the mere corrosion contribution in the synergistic damaging process. Differential experiments were carried out without and with the addition of 300 g L^{-1} of glass microspheres (Graziani s.r.l.), having a size of 200 ± 30 μm, representative of the erodent dimensions, hardness and mass relevant to the target application.

The experimental protocol was defined in view of ranking the three materials considered, in terms of their performance under erosion-corrosion resulting from abrasion by the slurry consisting of solid particles and a neutral, Cl$^-$-containing aqueous electrolyte. In order to place these results in context, other types of tests were performed for selected materials: erosion-corrosion caused by the impingement of the stirred aqueous solution and mere erosion with dry particles. Erosion conditions were defined by setting a rotation speed of 800 rpm and corrosion was controlled by applying a potential difference of 5 volts between the driving electrodes. All experiments were run for 18 h. In the slurry tests, we employed a mixture of 150 mL of electrolyte and 150 g of particles. In the experiments with the pure electrolyte and with the dry glass microspheres, the sample was contacted with 300 mL of liquid and 300 g of particulate, respectively.

The electrochemical measurements were performed using a PARSTAT 2273 potentiostat/galvanostat (Princeton Applied Research), controlled with "Power Corr" corrosion software. Weight losses were measured by a Sartorius weight balance with an accuracy of 10^{-4} g. The surface morphology of the samples was examined by scanning electron microscopy (SEM) with a EVO 40 instrument (Carl Zeiss AG, Jena, Germany).

3. Results

Two different coated systems and an uncoated reference material were chosen as the case study to prove the reliability of the proposed technique for studying erosion-corrosion problems. The morphology of the two coated systems (carbon steel coated with ENP and with Colmonoy 6) is reported in the SEM micrographs of Figure 2, where secondary electron (SE) and backscattered electrode (BSE) cross-sections are shown.

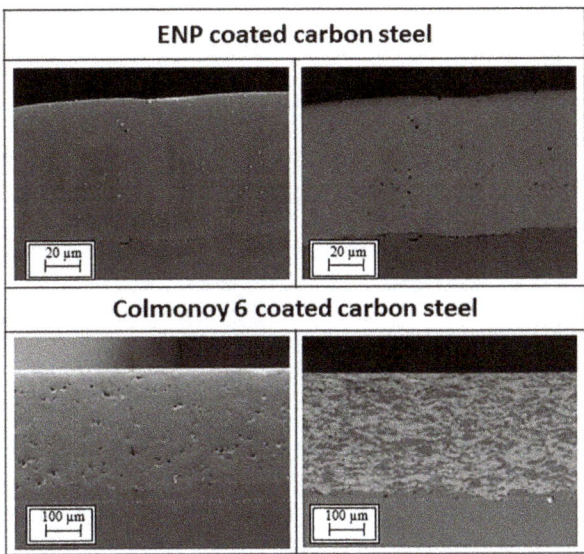

Figure 2. SE (**left**) and BSE (**right**) cross-sections of high phosphorus Electroless Nickel (ENP)-and Colmonoy 6-coated samples in pristine conditions.

ENP coating was dense and adherent to the substrate. Colmonoy 6 coating was a less dense layer, with some porosities, not interconnected, with a good adhesion to the substrate. BSE images allow us to better highlight the microstructure of Colmonoy 6, composed by a Nickel matrix with a dispersion of hard phases, mainly carbides. The signs of the final grinding process employed to get uniformity and pore closure are visible on the surface.

Figure 3 shows the chronoamperograms obtained during slurry erosion-corrosion testing for carbon steel specimens coated with ENP and Colmonoy 6 layers. It can be observed that, as expected, uncoated carbon steel was the most sensitive sample, yielding an average corrosion current density (c.d.) of 0.297 ± 0.006 mA cm^{-2}. The ENP coating imparts an appreciable degree of protection, resulting in a lower mean corrosion c.d. of 0.266 ± 0.007 mA cm^{-2}. Finally, the Colmonoy 6-coated sample was found to be notably more resistant, exhibiting a corrosion c.d. of 0.225 ± 0.007 mA cm^{-2}. In addition to the absolute values of the current density, reported above, that allow a global ranking of the erosion-corrosion performance of the different materials under the investigated conditions, their time trends yield some mechanistic information. Specifically, the different current density trends (increasing versus decreasing plots) observed in the initial part of the chronoamperograms can be explained by means of different model of passive film formation in analogy to what has been reported for hard metals [31]. A decreasing current trend denotes a tendency to improve passivation as erosion time lapses, this can be due to compaction of the pseudo-passivating corrosion product layer [31] or to plastic deformation of the underlying metal, resulting in lower metal activity [32]. In particular, this self-healing type of behavior can set in after an initial training period, as in the case of the Colmonoy 6 sample [33]. Finally, the increasing current density found with the ENP-coated sample after ca. 55,000 s, might denote incipient failure of the protective layer.

The weight loss measurements performed after the erosion-corrosion testing provided limited, but significant information. Indeed, with the uncoated and with the ENP-coated sample a weight loss of approximately 10 mg was measured. With the Colmonoy 6-coated sample, the mass loss was not appreciated. This result is consistent with what was observed by visual inspection of the samples (see below).

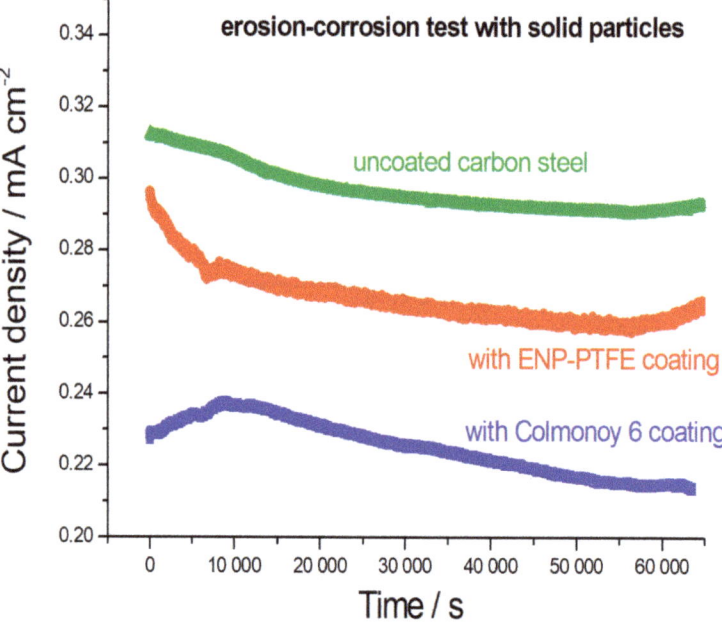

Figure 3. Chronoamperograms obtained with specimens of: uncoated carbon steel and the same carbon steel coated with ENP and Colmonoy 6, in a bipolar electrode configuration, during the erosion-corrosion test in the presence of eroding agent. A potential difference of 5 volts was applied between the driving electrodes for 18 h, imposing a rotation speed of 800 rpm to the specimens.

Figures 4 and 5 show macrographs and SEM micrographs of the samples tested for slurry erosion corrosion, compared with those taken with the same material in the pristine state. The images were taken on the front, back and a lateral surfaces to highlight the effects of the sample orientation with respect to the rotating shaft and the direction of rotation. In Figure 4, the uncoated specimen exhibits clear erosion marks, accompanied by the accumulation of corrosion products. The ENP-coated samples, instead, show a characteristic blackening of the surface as well as evident material removal, corresponding to the measured mass loss of ca. 10 mg. Specimens with the Colmonoy 6 coating are negligibly affected by the erosion-corrosion test, that causes only slight scratches.

The SEM micrographs of Figure 5 disclose that the uncoated carbon steel specimen undergoes both superficial and localized corrosion as a result of erosion-corrosion testing. The micrographs of ENP-coated specimens showed appreciable localized corrosion effects, together with notable material-removal marks. Colmonoy 6-coated samples show some pitting corrosion in correspondence of the erosion scratches.

The tests were completed by comparing the outcomes of erosion-corrosion testing with further damaging conditions that could highlight the peculiarities of each material. In the case of uncoated carbon steel, the least corrosion-resistant material, pure erosion conditions were also considered. Instead, in the case of the least erosion-corrosion coating, ENP, both pure corrosion and pure corrosion were considered in order to single out the individual impact of each factor. Figure 6 reports macrographs and micrographs of uncoated carbon steep subjected to pure erosion testing: evident signs left by the solid particulate are clearly observable, whereas the weight loss was negligible.

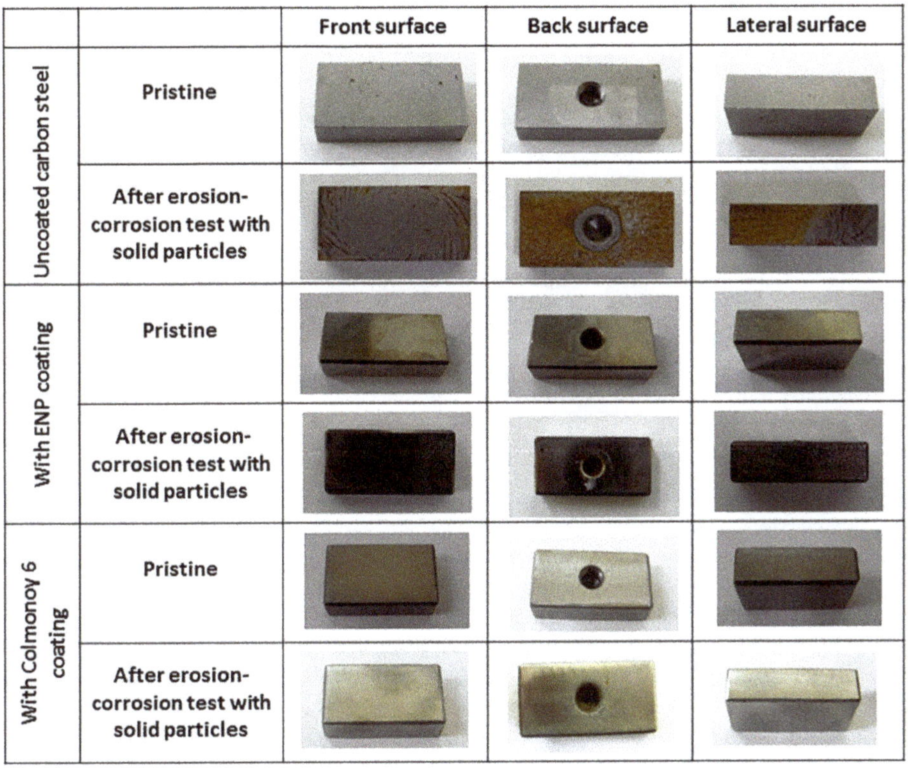

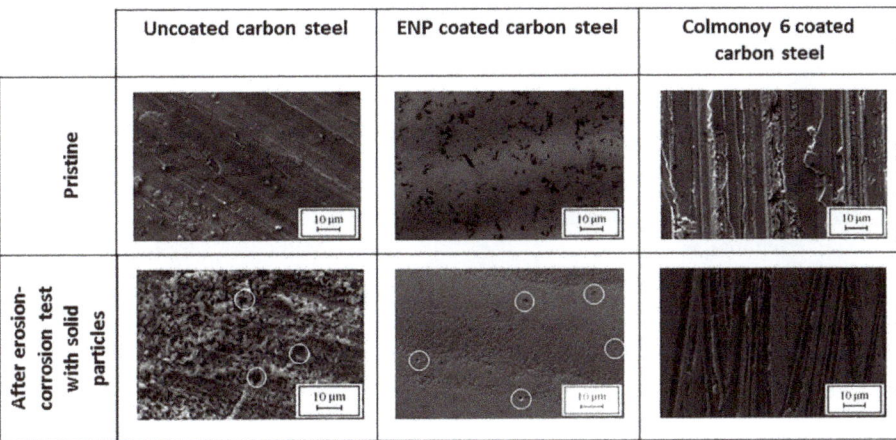

Figure 4. Macrographs of uncoated carbon steel samples and carbon steel coated with ENP and Colmonoy 6, in pristine conditions and after testing for slurry erosion-corrosion under the conditions specified in Figure 2.

Figure 5. Scanning electron micrographs (SEM) of uncoated carbon steel samples and carbon steel coated with ENP and Colmonoy 6, in pristine conditions and after testing for slurry erosion-corrosion under the conditions specified in Figure 3. The most evident pits have been marked with white circles.

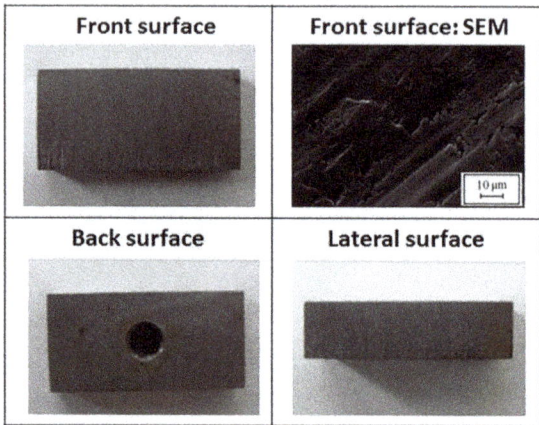

Figure 6. Macrographs and SEM micrograph of the carbon steel sample after testing for erosion with dry glass microspheres.

In Figure 7A, we show chronoamperogram of the ENP-coated sample tested under erosion-corrosion conditions caused by electrolyte impingement without particulate suspension. Comparing these results with those of Figure 3, it can be observed that the average corrosion c.d. in the slurry test was more than five times higher than that observed in the solution without eroding agent (0.052 ± 0.004 mA cm^{-2}), thus allowing us to single out the synergy of the two damaging processes. Figure 7B shows that pure erosion testing gives rise to material removal, in particular on the lateral surfaces, while the electrolyte impingement test gives rise to blackening effects on the edges, similar to those found with the slurry test. The micrographs of Figure 7C disclose appreciable localized corrosion effects resulting from the electrolyte-impingement test, while pure erosion gives rise to evident surface scratching. No appreciable weight loss was measured in these cases.

The above-reported erosion-corrosion tests thus allowed us to clearly determine the erosion-corrosion resistance ranking of the investigated materials. Specifically, we found that the Colmonoy 6 coating imparts the best erosion-corrosion performance under the investigated conditions while the ENP coating worsens the performance of the surface of the material, with respect to uncoated conditions, owing to enhanced localized corrosion. Indeed, on the basis of the analysis performed by evaluating the weight loss and the electrochemical and morphological differences observed between the cases of mere erosion or corrosion in the absence of sand and the case of erosion-corrosion, we noticed a high synergic effect both for uncoated carbon steel and for ENP-coated samples. In detail, in the case of the uncoated sample, the weight loss was negligible after the pure erosion test, whereas a weight loss of 10 mg was measured as a result of the erosion-corrosion test. In the case of ENP-coated sample, the average corrosion current density in the slurry test was five times higher than that observed in the solution without an eroding agent. The Colmonoy 6-coated specimen presented negligible damages after the erosion-corrosion test.

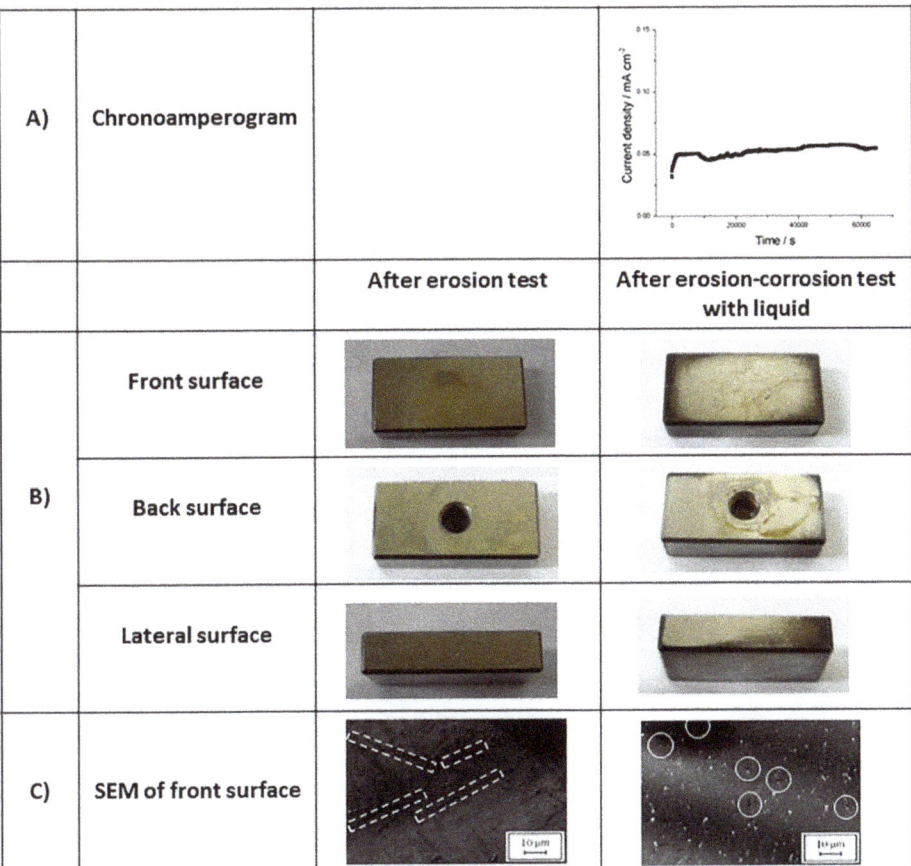

Figure 7. Erosion and erosion-corrosion test results for ENP-coated carbon steel. (**A**) Chronoamperograms recorded during electrolyte-impingement testing. A potential difference of 5 volts was applied between the driving electrodes for 18 h, imposing a rotation speed of 800 rpm to the specimens. (**B**) Macrographs. (**C**) SEM micrographs. The most evident pits have been marked with solid white circles, the most evident scratches have been marked with dashed white rectangles.

4. Conclusions

Bipolar electrochemistry was applied for the first time to an erosion-corrosion investigation of coated metallic samples. The effects due to the erosion-corrosion by solid particles and fluid and those due to simple erosion were evaluated and distinguished. A resistance ranking of the investigated materials was clearly determined. Their performances were correlated with the characteristics of the coatings. From slurry erosion-corrosion testing, a mass loss of 10 mg was evaluated for the ENP-coated specimen, together with blackening of the surface, whereas it was negligible for the Colmonoy 6-coated sample. Moreover, the Colmonoy 6-coated sample was found to be more resistant than the ENP-coated one, both in terms of corrosion current density and in terms of observed surface damages. The higher erosion-corrosion resistance of Colmonoy 6 with respect to the ENP-coated sample observed in study could be related to the difference in the chemical composition and in the thickness of the coatings, combined with the lower roughness and the higher microhardness of Colmonoy 6.

Finally, the feasibility of this contactless approach proved the possibility to perform experiments on coated samples subject to erosion and corrosion processes, thus notably extending the scope of erosion-corrosion testing under electrochemical control.

Author Contributions: Conceptualization, C.M. and B.B.; Methodology, C.M. and B.B.; Experimental activity C.M.; Data Curation, C.M., F.L. and B.B.; Writing, Review and Editing, C.M., F.L. and B.B.; Supervision, B.B.; Funding Acquisition, C.M. and B.B. All authors have read and agree to the published version of the manuscript.

Funding: The research leading to these results has received funding from Italian National Operative Programme (PON) for Research and Competitiveness 2007–2013.

Acknowledgments: The authors would like to thank General Electric, corporate partner of the project and, in particular, Domenico Di Pietro and Paolo Guastamacchia, for providing the samples used in the tests and their surface properties.

Conflicts of Interest: The authors declare no conflict of interest. The funders had no role in the design of the study; in the collection, analyses, or interpretation of data; in the writing of the manuscript, or in the decision to publish the results.

References

1. Lu, B. Erosion-corrosion in oil and gas production. *Res. Rev. Mater. Sci. Chem.* **2013**, *2*, 19–60.
2. Okonkwo, P.C.; Mohamed, A.M.A. Erosion-corrosion in oil and gas industry: A review. *Int. J. Metall. Mater. Sci. Eng.* **2014**, *4*, 7–28.
3. Shirazi, S.A.; Mclaury, B.S.; Shadley, J.R.; Roberts, K.P.; Rybicki, E.F.; Rincon, H.E.; Hassani, S.; Al-Mutahar, F.M.; Al-Aithan, G.H. Erosion–corrosion in oil and gas pipelines. *Oil Gas Pipelines* **2015**, 399–422. [CrossRef]
4. Smith, L. Control of corrosion in oil and gas production tubing. *Br. Corros. J.* **1999**, *34*, 247–253. [CrossRef]
5. Mele, C.; Boniardi, M.V.; Casaroli, A.; Degli Esposti, M.; Di Pietro, D.; Guastamacchia, P.; Bozzini, B. A comprehensive assessment of the performance of corrosion resistant alloys in hot acidic brines for application in oil and gas production. *Corros. Eng. Sci. Technol.* **2017**, *52*, 99–113. [CrossRef]
6. Kawahara, Y. An overview on corrosion-resistant coating technologies in biomass/waste-to-energy plants in recent decades. *Coatings* **2016**, *6*, 34. [CrossRef]
7. Reyes, M.; Neville, A. Degradation mechanisms of Co-based alloy and WC metal–matrix composites for drilling tools offshore. *Wear* **2003**, *255*, 1143–1156. [CrossRef]
8. El Rayes, M.M.; Abdo, H.S.; Khalil, K.A. Erosion-corrosion of cermet coating. *Int. J. Electrochem. Sci.* **2013**, *8*, 1117–1137.
9. Oksa, M.; Metsäjoki, J.; Kärki, J. Corrosion testing of thermal spray coatings in a biomass co-firing power plant. *Coatings* **2016**, *6*, 65. [CrossRef]
10. De Souza, V.A.; Neville, A. Corrosion and erosion damage mechanisms during erosion–corrosion of WC–Co–Cr cermet coatings. *Wear* **2003**, *255*, 146–156. [CrossRef]
11. Souza, V.A.D.; Neville, A. Corrosion and synergy in a WCCoCr HVOF thermal spray coating—Understanding their role in erosion–corrosion degradation. *Wear* **2005**, *259*, 171–180. [CrossRef]
12. Levy, A.V. The erosion-corrosion behavior of protective coatings. *Surf. Coat. Technol.* **1988**, *36*, 387–406. [CrossRef]
13. Espallargas, N.; Berget, J.; Guilemany, J.M.; Benedetti, A.V.; Suegama, P.H. Cr3C2–NiCr and WC–Ni thermal spray coatings as alternatives to hard chromium for erosion–corrosion resistance. *Surf. Coat. Technol.* **2008**, *202*, 1405–1417. [CrossRef]
14. Stack, M.M.; Jana, B.D.; Abdelrahman, S.M. Models and mechanisms of erosion–corrosion in metals. In *Tribocorrosion of Passive Metals and Coatings*; Elsevier, Woodhead Publishing: Cambridge, UK, 2011; pp. 153e–187e.
15. Tiwari, A.; Seman, S.; Singh, G.; Jayaganthan, R. Nanocrystalline cermet coatings for erosion-corrosion protection. *Coatings* **2019**, *9*, 400. [CrossRef]
16. Postlethwaite, J.; Nesic, S. Erosion-corrosion in single and multiphase flow. In *Uhlig's Corrosion Handbook*, 2nd ed.; Revie, W., Ed.; John Wiley & Sons, Inc.: New York, NY, USA, 2000; pp. 249–272.
17. Wood, R.J.K. Erosion-corrosion interactions and their effects on marine and offshore materials. *Wear* **2006**, *261*, 1012–1023. [CrossRef]

18. López, D.M.; Falleiros, N.A.; Tschiptschin, A.P. Use of electrochemical tests for assessment of the effect of erosive particle size on the erosion-corrosion behaviour of AISI 304L austenitic stainless steel. *Mater. Res.* **2016**, *19*, 451–458. [CrossRef]
19. Pitt, C.H.; Chang, Y.M. Jet slurry corrosive wear of high-chromium cast iron and high-carbon steel grinding ball alloys. *Corrosion* **1986**, *42*, 312–317. [CrossRef]
20. Hu, X.; Neville, A. The electrochemical response of stainless steels in liquid–solid impingement. *Wear* **2005**, *258*, 641–648. [CrossRef]
21. Xu, Y.; Luo, J.L.; Tan, M.Y. An overview of techniques for measuring the interaction between erosion and corrosion. *Corros. Prev.* **2017**, *99*, 1–13.
22. Fosdick, S.E.; Knust, K.N.; Scida, K.; Crooks, R.M. Bipolar electrochemistry. *Angew. Chem. Int. Ed.* **2013**, *52*, 10438–10456. [CrossRef]
23. Crooks, R.M. Principles of bipolar electrochemistry. *Chem. ElectroChem.* **2016**, *3*, 357–359. [CrossRef]
24. Kuhn, A.; Crooks, R.M.; Inagi, S. A compelling case for bipolar electrochemistry. *Chem. ElectroChem* **2016**, *3*, 351–352. [CrossRef]
25. Koefoed, L.; Pedersen, S.U.; Daasbjerg, K. Bipolar electrochemistry—A wireless approach for electrode reactions. *Curr. Opin. Electrochem.* **2017**, *2*, 13–17. [CrossRef]
26. Loget, G.; Zigah, D.; Bouffier, L.; Sojic, N.; Kuhn, A. Bipolar electrochemistry: From materials science to motion and beyond. *Acc. Chem. Res.* **2013**, *46*, 2513–2523. [CrossRef] [PubMed]
27. Sequeira, C.A.C.; Cardoso, D.S.P.; Gameiro, M.L.F. Bipolar electrochemistry, a focal point of future research. *Chem. Eng. Commun.* **2016**, *203*, 1001–1008. [CrossRef]
28. Phuakkong, O.; Sentic, M.; Li, H.; Warakulwit, C.; Limtrakul, J.; Sojic, N.; Kuhn, A.; Ravaine, V.; Zigah, D. Wireless synthesis and activation of electrochemiluminescent thermoresponsive janus objects using bipolar electrochemistry. *Langmuir* **2016**, *32*, 12995–13002. [CrossRef]
29. Munktell, S.; Tydén, M.; Högström, J.; Nyholm, L.; Björefors, F. Bipolar electrochemistry for high-throughput corrosion screening. *Electrochem. Commun.* **2013**, *34*, 274–277. [CrossRef]
30. Saeed, A. Application of Bipolar Electrochemistry for Corrosion Screening of Type 420 Stainless Steel in Sodium Chloride Solution. Master's Thesis, School of Materials Corrosion and Protection Centre, University of Manchester, Manchester, UK, 2017.
31. De Gaudenzi, G.P.; Bozzini, B. Meccanismi di corrosione del metallo duro. *La Metall. Ital.* **2017**, *11–12*, 39–49.
32. Bozzini, B.; Ricotti, M.E.; Boniardi, M.; Mele, C. Evaluation of erosion–corrosion in multiphase flow via CFD and experimental analysis. *Wear* **2003**, *255*, 237–245. [CrossRef]
33. De Gaudenzi, G.P.; Tedeschi, S.; Mele, C.; Bozzini, B. The effect of binder composition on the tribo-corrosion behavior of cemented carbides in simulated tertaphasic flows. In Proceedings of the Euro PM2018 Congress, Bilbao, Spain, 14–18 October 2018; Paper 3390848.

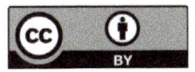

© 2020 by the authors. Licensee MDPI, Basel, Switzerland. This article is an open access article distributed under the terms and conditions of the Creative Commons Attribution (CC BY) license (http://creativecommons.org/licenses/by/4.0/).

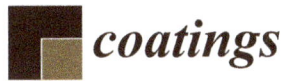

Article

Surface Morphological Features of Molybdenum Irradiated by a Single Laser Pulse

Roberto Montanari *, Ekaterina Pakhomova, Riccardo Rossi, Maria Richetta and Alessandra Varone

Department of Industrial Engineering, University of Rome "Tor Vergata", 00133 Rome, Italy; pakhomovaea@mail.ru (E.P.); r.rossi@ing.uniroma2.it (R.R.); richetta@uniroma2.it (M.R.); alessandra.varone@uniroma2.it (A.V.)
* Correspondence: roberto.montanari@uniroma2.it; Tel.: +39-6-7259-7182

Received: 19 December 2019; Accepted: 9 January 2020; Published: 11 January 2020

Abstract: Molybdenum (Mo) is considered a plasma facing material alternative to tungsten (W) for manufacturing the divertor armours of International Thermonuclear Experimental Reactor (ITER). Transient thermal loads of high energy occurring in a tokamak during the service life have been simulated through a single laser pulse delivered by a Nd:YAG/Glass laser, and the effects have then been examined through scanning electron microscopy (SEM) observations. An erosion crater forms in correspondence with the laser spot due to the vaporization and melting of the metal, while all around a network of cracks induced by thermal stresses is observed. The findings have been compared to results of similar experiments on W and literature data. The morphology of the crater and the surrounding area is different from that of W: the crater is larger and shallower in the case of Mo, while its walls are characterized by long filaments, not observed in W, because the lower viscosity and surface tension of Mo allow an easier flow of the liquid metal. Most importantly, the volume of Mo ablated from the surface by the single laser pulse is about ten times that of W. This critical aspect is of particular relevance and leads us to conclude that W remains the best solution for manufacturing the armours of the ITER divertor.

Keywords: molybdenum; nuclear fusion reactors; laser; surface damage; microstructure

1. Introduction

Plasma facing materials (PFM) of future nuclear fusion reactors will be exposed, in addition to a steady state heat flux, to transient events of high energy such as disruption, edge localized modes (ELM), and vertical displacement events (VDE). The large heat fluxes occurring during transient events induced by plasma instabilities may lead to the melting and vaporization of PFMs with the consequent contamination of plasma and the damage of PFM components.

At present, tungsten (W) and W-1%La_2O_3 alloy are the most promising materials for manufacturing the divertor armours of ITER [1–5]. W has the highest melting point of all metals and exhibits excellent thermo-mechanical characteristics, a low sputtering rate, and a tritium inventory; therefore, thin W coatings on graphite and carbon fibre composites have already been adopted in reactors like JET [5] and ASDEX-U [6]. The drawbacks of W are the poor machinability at an ambient temperature and the high ductile-to-brittle transition temperature. Moreover, the resistance to thermal shocks during ELMs is also a matter of concern [7] because a fibrous nanostructure forms on the W surface due to low-energy He ion irradiation with detrimental effects on the thermo-mechanical properties [8].

The dispersion of La_2O_3 particles in the W matrix improves the toughness [9], enhances the resistance to thermal shocks and creep, increases the recrystallization temperature, and hinders grain growth at a high temperature (up to ~1750 °C).

Some studies were also carried out to assess the effects of the dispersion in W of other oxides (Y_2O_3, TiO, etc.) or other elements (Ta, Ti), with controversial results [10,11]. In fact, some properties resulted in being improved; however, the added components often involve the generation of W dust into plasma; thus, as of now, all the required conditions to develop a reliable divertor armour have not been satisfied.

Recently, molybdenum (Mo) has attracted increasing interest as a possible PFM alternative to W [12–16]. As shown in Table 1, Mo is a high-Z refractory metal with very good physical properties (density, melting point, boiling point, and thermal conductivity), even if it is a little inferior to W. On the contrary, the ductile to brittle transition temperature (DBTT) of Mo is much lower, and it exhibits a better resistance to thermal shocks [15–17].

Table 1. A comparison of some physical properties of W and Mo: atomic number Z, density ρ_A, melting point T_M, boiling point T_B, thermal conductivity ξ, ductile to brittle transition temperature DBTT, latent heat of fusion E_M, and latent heat of vaporization E_V.

Metal	Z	ρ_A at 20 °C [g·cm^{-3}]	T_M [°C]	T_B [°C]	ξ [W·m^{-1}·K^{-1}]	DBTT [°C]	E_M [kJ·mole^{-1}]	E_V [kJ·mole^{-1}]
W	74	19.25	3422	5555	110	+400	35.4	824
Mo	42	10.22	2623	4639	142	−20	32	598

Another relevant advantage of Mo to W is its behavior under prolonged irradiation by 14 MeV neutrons of a fusion power plant. W transmutes to osmium (Os) via rhenium (Re) and forms the W–Os–Re alloy. Cottrell [18] calculated that five years in a fusion power plant will have transmuted pure W into an alloy of about 75 (at.%) W, 13 (at.%) Os, and 12 (at.%) Re, a composition close to that of the brittle σ phase. In the same irradiation conditions, Mo would produce 1.1% Tc and 0.65% Ru after 5 years, well inside the primary Mo phase field at 1500 °C.

The erosion/redeposition characteristics of pure Mo and W are similar [19], but the fractional hydrogen isotope retention is lower in Mo than in W [20].

In this work the specific conditions of transient events have been simulated by irradiating Mo samples through a Nd:YAG/Glass high power laser source, suitable to release a high thermal load in a very short time (~15 ns) on a small area (~200 μm) and to reach a surface power density on the focal plane of about 1.7×10^{12} W·cm^{-2}.

The effects of the laser pulse on the sample surface have been then investigated through 3D surface analysis and scanning electron microscopy (SEM) observations. The same experimental procedure was adopted in previous works of present authors to study the behavior of W (bulk and plasma sprayed) [21,22] and W-1%La_2O_3 alloy [23]. The results are discussed in comparison to those previously obtained by us on W, the principal candidate material for building the armours of ITER, and in general to literature data. A recent critical overview about material erosion of candidate materials like W and Mo is reported in [24].

2. Material and Experimental Section

2.1. Sample Characteristics

The material (purity of 99.9 wt.%) examined in the present work was supplied by PLANSEE (Metallwerk Plansee, Reutte, Austria) in the form of plates with a thickness of 25 mm, which were cut to obtain samples with dimensions of 25 mm × 20 mm (Figure 1a).

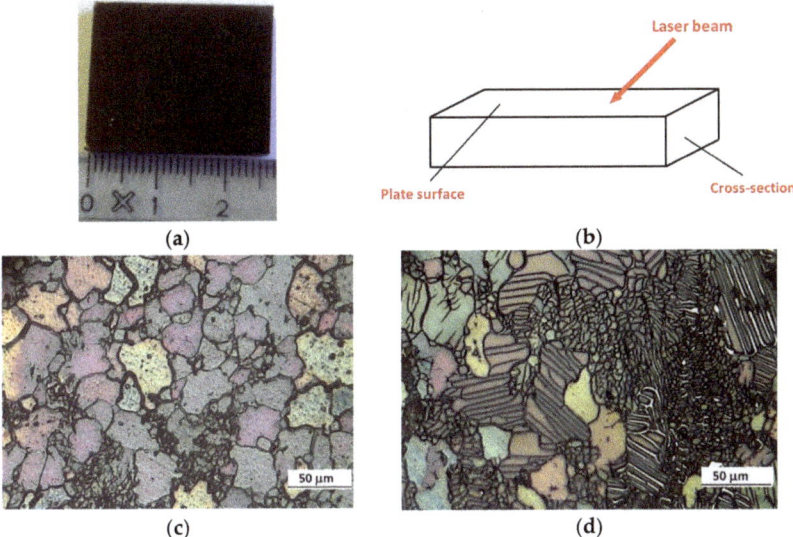

Figure 1. Picture(**a**) and (**b**) sketch of the sample. The structure of the examined Mo samples: plate surface (**c**), cross-section (**d**).

The structure of Mo grains on the plate surface and in the cross-section (Figure 1b) has been examined through light microscopy. After conventional metallographic surface preparation, the sample has been etched by immersion for 60 s in a boiling solution of H_2O 100 mL with H_2O_2 (30%) 1 mL, and observed by using an optical microscope (Union Optical Co., Ltd., Tokyo, Japan).

Figure 1c,d shows how the grain structure is different on the plate surface (c) and in the cross-section (d). A large part of the plate surface is covered by grains with a mean size D of about 40 µm, while some zones exhibit smaller grains of about 5 µm (Figure 1b). In the cross-section, small grains (~5 µm) are the dominant feature, and only few grains of larger size are present and show elongated substructures.

The Mo samples were then characterized through X-ray diffraction (XRD, diffractometer Philips, Eindhoven, The Netherlands). Figure 2 displays the XRD pattern obtained by focusing the beam on the plate surface.

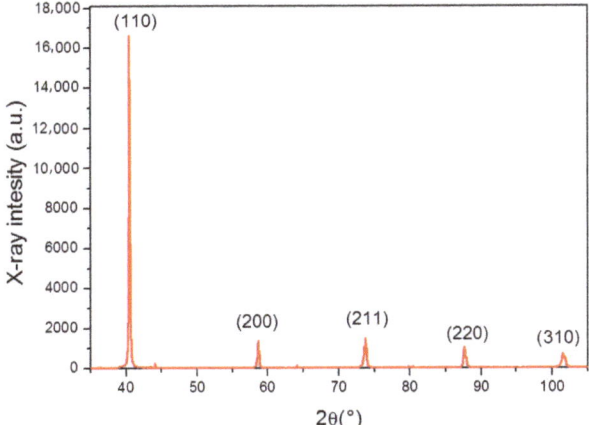

Figure 2. The XRD pattern of the examined Mo.

The XRD pattern displayed in Figure 2 was collected by operating in a step-scanning mode with Cu-Kα radiation (wavelength λ = 0.1508 nm), 2θ steps of 0.05°, and a counting time of 5 s per step. To assess the possible presence of preferred grain orientations, the relative intensities of the main reflections have been compared to those reported in the JCPDS-ICDD database [25], file 42-1120, and corresponding to a material with random oriented grains. The results displayed in Table 2 show that Mo used in the present experiments exhibits a strong {110} texture.

Table 2. A comparison of the intensities of main reflections to those reported in the JCPDS-ICDD database.

Miller Index {hkl}	110	200	211	220	310
JCPDS-ICDD	100	16	31	9	14
Sample	100	8	9	6	4

To determine the cell parameter and the dislocation density, high precision peak profiles were recorded with 2θ steps of 0.005° and a counting time of 5 s per step. The cell parameter a resulted in 0.3150 nm, very close to the value of 0.3147 nm given by the JCPDS-ICDD database.

The dislocation density ρ has been determined from the line broadening of XRD peak profiles. The total line broadening β_T of a peak is the sum of two contributions due to the size D of coherently diffracting domains (β_D), namely the grains, and to the micro-strains ε (β_ε):

$$\beta_T = \beta_D + \beta_\varepsilon = \frac{K\lambda}{D\cos\theta} + 2\varepsilon \tan\theta \quad (1)$$

θ being the Bragg angle and K = 0.89. Since the mean D value is ~10 μm, β_D is negligible and $\beta_T \cong \beta_\varepsilon$. The dislocation density ρ has then been calculated using the Williamson-Smallman relationship [26]:

$$\rho = \Xi\varepsilon^2/k_0 b^2 \quad (2)$$

where Ξ = 16.1 and $k_0 \cong 1$ are constants, and b = 0.18186 nm is the modulus of Burgers vector. The dislocation density ρ resulted in 2.0×10^{10} cm^{-2}.

The samples were also submitted to Vickers micro-hardness tests (Shimadzu corporation, Kyoto, Japan). The mean value obtained from 20 tests (300 g, 10 s) was 211 ± 5 HV. The yield stress σ_Y = 540 MPa was determined from the FIMEC test [27].

2.2. Laser Source

The plate surface of the Mo samples have been irradiated (see Figure 1) by a single laser pulse delivered by the laser system—Tor Vergata Laser-Plasma Source (TVLPS) [28], a no-commercial device which consists of a Nd:YAG oscillator, based on the Q-switched technique, followed by four amplification stages. The first two are also Nd:YAG, while the last ones are Nd:Glass. The pulse parameters of the present experiments are: wavelength λ = 1064 nm, pulse duration Δτ ≈ 15 ns, pulse energy E_p ≈ 8 J, Transverse Electromagnetical Mode is TEM00, P-polarized, focal spot size Φ = 200 μm, and surface power density on the focal plane I = 1.7×10^{12} W·cm^{-2}. The plasma electronic temperature at the critical surface ($T_e \approx 1.218 \times 10^6$ K) simulates the conditions of transient events occurring in a tokamak due to plasma instability.

The experiments were carried out in a vacuum chamber ($P \approx 10^{-5}$ bar), and the laser beam hits the samples with an incidence angle of 45° to minimize debris projection near the target. More details about the experimental set-up are reported in previous works [21–23] on W (bulk and plasma sprayed) and W-1%La$_2$O$_3$ alloy, which were irradiated in the same conditions.

A spectrometer USB 2000 model (Ocean Optics, 4301 Metric Drive, Winter Park, FL, USA) was used to collect the spectrum from plasma induced by a laser pulse.

After laser irradiation, the surface morphological changes of the Mo samples were studied through SEM observations (Hitachi SU70, Hitachi, Tokyo, Japan). A 3D surface analyzer (TalySurf CLI 2000, Taylor Hobson, Leicester, UK) was used to get level profiles in the zone hit by the laser spot.

3. Results and Discussion

Figure 3 displays the spectrum recorded from plasma induced by a laser pulse through the spectrometer USB 2000. It only exhibits the lines of Mo, whereas those of other metals are not present. Some lines of low intensity corresponding to O are also detected and can be attributed to native oxide on the sample surface.

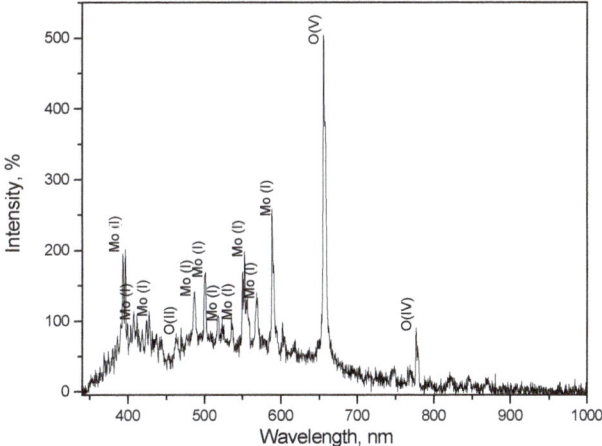

Figure 3. Spectrum recorded from plasma induced by a laser pulse (wavelengths from 250 to 1000 nm).

The zone on the sample surface affected by laser pulse irradiation is almost circular with a diameter of ~2.2 mm (Figure 4), i.e., much larger than that of the laser spot ($\Phi = 200$ µm).

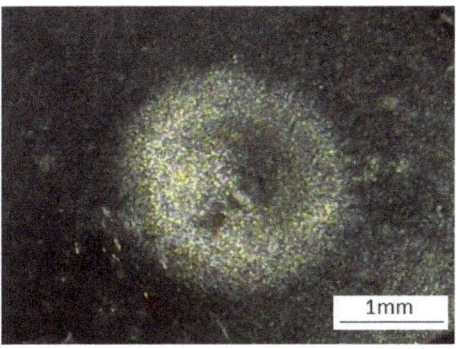

Figure 4. The surface zone affected by the laser pulse.

As shown in the SEM micrographs of Figure 5, an erosion crater with a diameter of ~300 µm (a) forms in the central area of the laser spot where the beam has the highest intensity. The laser intensity has a Gaussian shape; thus, its maximum is at the centre, and it radially decreases toward the periphery. The larger fraction of the energy is released in the central part of the spot, causing the melting and vaporization of the metal; the crater formation is due to the ejection of part of the molten metal. Figure 5b displays a drop of the ejected metal fallen and re-solidified in a zone near the crater. Sinclair et al. [16] demonstrated that the surface melting of Mo begins when the energy density reaches a value of ~1.0 MJ·m^{-2} and that the droplet formation and boiling starts from ~1.4 MJ·m^{-2}, namely values much lower than those involved in the present experiments.

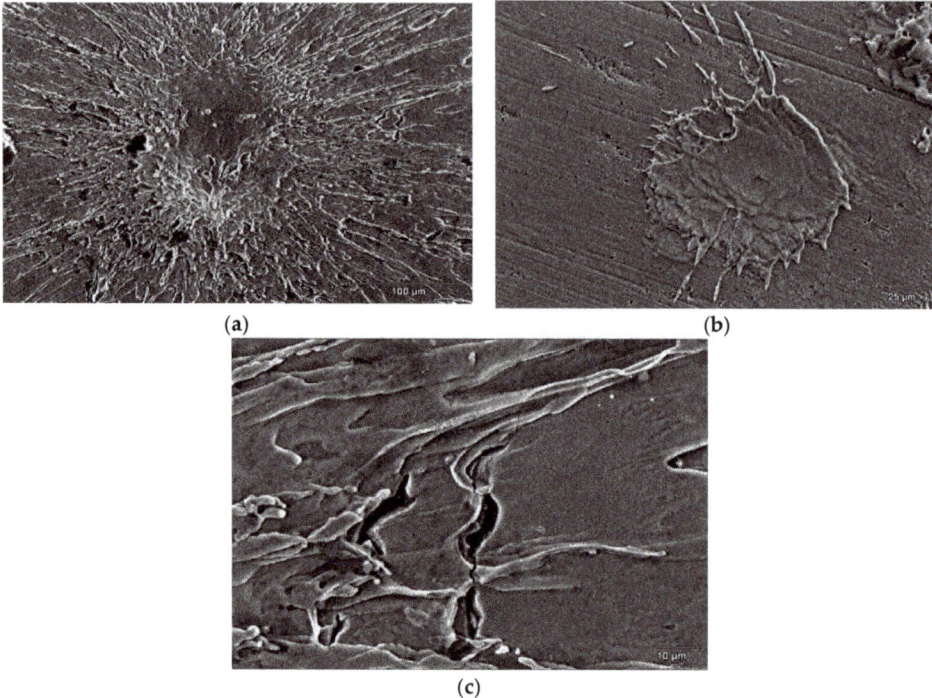

Figure 5. SEM micrographs displaying the zone irradiated by the laser pulse: (**a**) the crater; (**b**) the splash of molten metal ejected from the crater; and (**c**) a detail of the crater at a higher magnification showing some cracks.

Another effect resulting from the Gaussian intensity profile of the spot is the occurrence of a temperature gradient in molten metal leading to a liquid movement along the radial direction, giving rise to the typical morphology of crater walls shown in the detail of Figure 5c and to the formation of a ridge around the crater. The crater walls are decorated by radially oriented filaments that are produced by the movement and successive solidification of the liquid metal.

The thermal stresses arising from the rapid heating and successive cooling of the external zone of the crater lead to the nucleation and growth of cracks like those shown in Figure 5c.

The morphology of the area affected by the laser pulse has been recorded through a 3D surface analyzer (see Figure 6a), and 10 level profiles of the crater, such as that displayed in Figure 6b, have been measured along different directions. The mean diameter and depth was 300 ± 9 and 17 ± 2 µm, respectively; thus, the aspect ratio of the crater (depth/diameter) is ~0.05666. The shape of the crater is quite different from that produced in W under the same experimental conditions (crater diameter = 75 µm, depth = 25 µm, and aspect ratio ~0.333 [21]), namely in the case of Mo it is larger and shallower. Such difference can be explained by considering the specific microstructure of the examined Mo and W samples and its relation with the thermal conductivity affecting the heat flow through the materials. Since the correlation between incoming and outgoing phonons is destroyed by the scattering occurring at an interface like a grain boundary [29,30], the thermal conductivity C decreases with the decreasing grain size d and can be written as:

$$C = \frac{C_0}{1 + \frac{R_K C_0}{d}} \qquad (3)$$

where C_0 is the grain interior thermal conductivity and R_K is the Kapitza resistance that measures the interface resistance to the thermal flow [31,32].

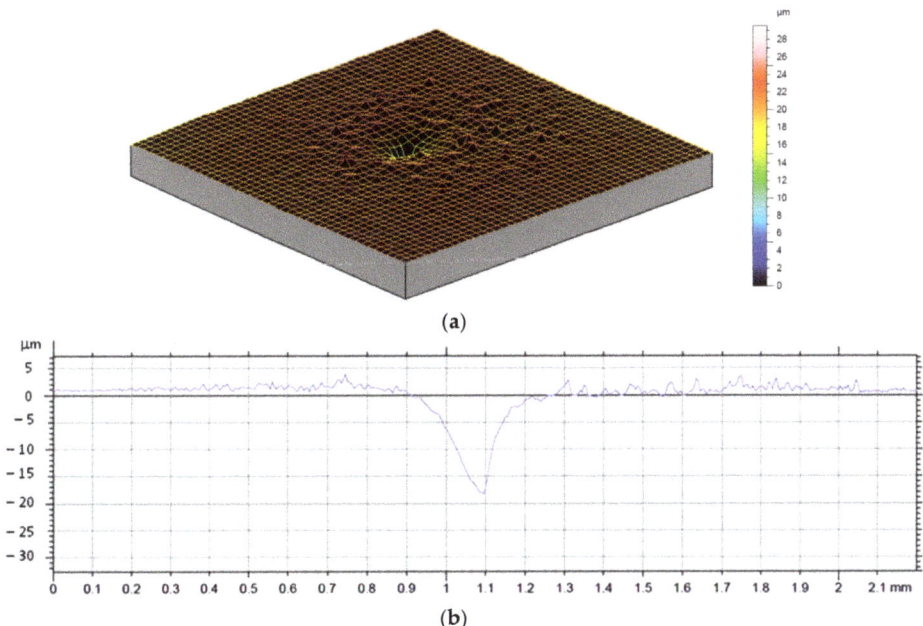

Figure 6. (a) The morphology of the laser irradiated zone measured through a 3D surface analyzer. A level profile of the crater determined from the image in (a) is displayed in (b).

W has equiaxed grains; thus, there is not a preferred direction for the heat flow, as a result of which the crater diameter and depth are comparable. On the contrary, in the case of Mo, heat moves easier along the surface than in the perpendicular direction because it encounters a lower number of interfaces (see Figure 1b,c), giving rise to a larger and shallower crater.

However, the most important difference between the behaviour of the two refractory metals regards the volume of material ablated from the surface by the single laser pulse. A rough estimation of such a volume has been made by considering the crater like a cone. From this calculation, the ablated volume in the case of Mo is about ten times that of W. This strictly depends on the latent heat of fusion E_M and latent heat of vaporization E_V of W, which are remarkably higher than those of Mo (see Table 1).

After melting, the liquid metal is flushed to the periphery, and its viscosity and surface tension determine the morphological features of the crater and surrounding zones, which are different from those of W because in that case [21,22] solidified drops decorating the crater walls have been observed but the long filaments displayed by Mo have not (see Figure 5).

The surface tension of Mo, determined by Paradis et al. [33] through the oscillation drop technique in conjunction with a vacuum electrostatic levitation furnace, can be expressed as:

$$\sigma(T) = 2.29 \times 10^3 - 0.26(T - T_m) \text{ (mN·m}^{-1}) \qquad (4)$$

while that of W is [34]:

$$\sigma(T) = 2.48 \times 10^3 - 0.31(T - T_m) \text{ (mN·m}^{-1}) \tag{5}$$

The surface tension values of molten Mo and W vs. temperature, calculated according to Equations (4) and (5), are plotted in Figure 7.

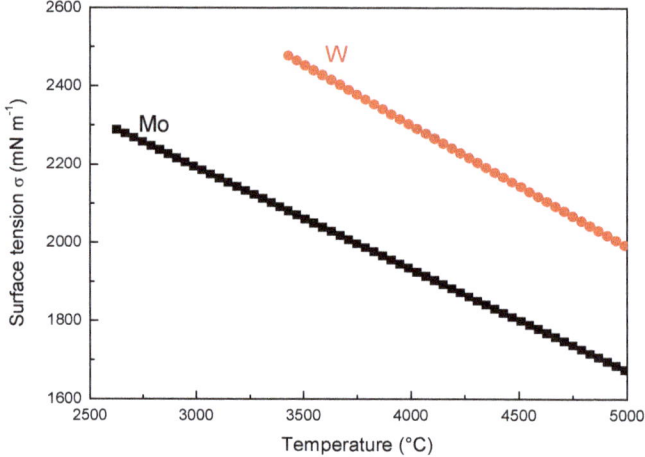

Figure 7. Surface tension of W and Mo vs. temperature, calculated according to the relationships of Paradis et al. [33,34].

The viscosity trends of liquid Mo [33–35] and W [36] vs. temperature are given by the Equations (6) and (7), respectively, and are plotted in Figure 8.

$$\eta(T) = 0.27\exp[73 \times 10^3/RT] \text{ (mPa·s)} \tag{6}$$

$$\eta(T) = 0.16\exp[3.9713 T_M/T] \text{ (mPa·s)} \tag{7}$$

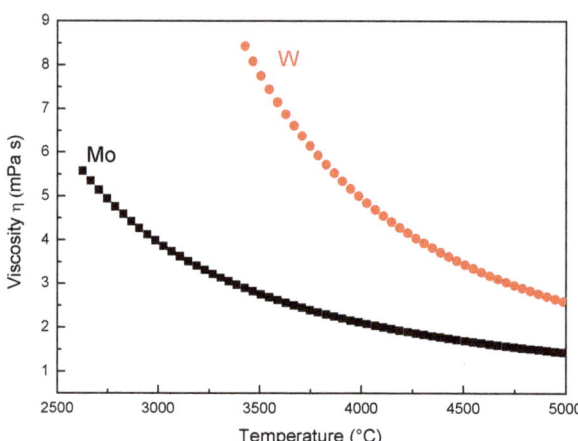

Figure 8. Viscosity of W and Mo vs. temperature, calculated according to Equations (5) and (6).

On these grounds, it is clear that the lower viscosity of Mo allows an easier flow of the liquid metal, leading to the formation of long filaments (see Figure 5) that are not observed in the case of W.

In a more external region outside the crater, from 300 μm to ~1 mm, the material exhibits bubbles like those shown in Figure 9a,b and long cracks. Such cracks are due to thermal stresses occurring in the metal after fast heating and successive cooling; as shown in Figure 9c, they depart from the bubbles to then propagate through the material. Similar results have been recently published by Straus et al. [37], who studied the damage of W and Mo surfaces induced by an ultraviolet laser radiation (λ ~ 47 nm).

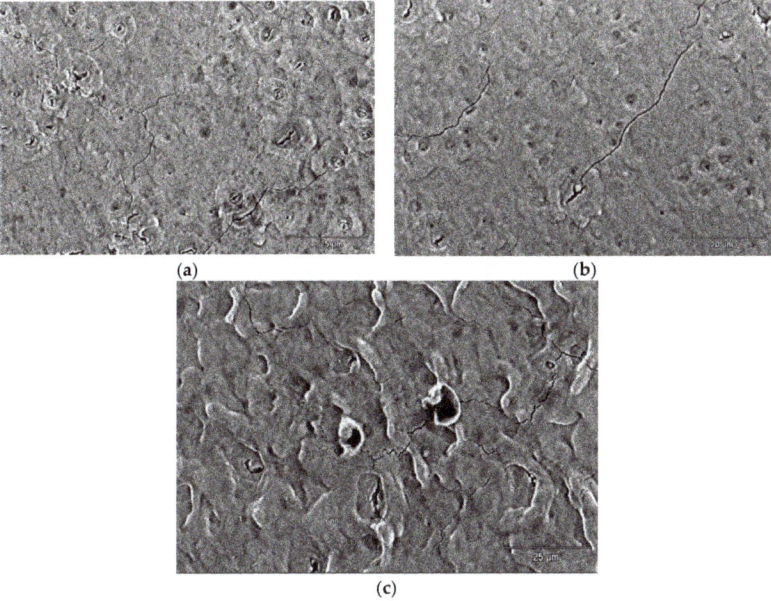

Figure 9. (a–c) The zone around the crater exhibits bubbles and long cracks often departing from the bubbles.

Figure 10a shows a cross-section of the crater: the morphology and size of the grains differs remarkably from that of the unaffected material (Figure 1c), since elongated substructures substantially disappeared, and grains with a size of a few microns cover only a small part of the observed area. The change can be explained by the grain growth induced by the strong heating in the zone close to where the melting occurs. The same phenomenon is also observed in Figure 10b, taken from a zone below the crater at a distance of about 500 μm from the sample surface, even if in this case the effect is limited because the larger distance involves a lower temperature increase.

Finally, no microstructural change has been detected at a distance of about 1 mm.

In future work, research will be focused on the regimes of high-energy exposure in order to explore the effects of different thermal loads. Treatments suitable for improving the structure and mechanical properties of Mo will also be investigated in order to get better behaviour under laser irradiation and to eliminate surface cracking. Another aspect that deserves to be deeply examined is the role of the original sample roughness, which can affect the erosion as well as tritium retention (e.g., see the paper of Eksaeva et al. [38]). However, the most critical aspect evidenced by the present experiments, namely the large volume ablated from the surface by the single laser pulse (~ten times that of W), seems difficult to resolve because the latent heat of fusion and latent heat of vaporization are intrinsic properties of the material and are not easily modifiable. On these grounds, W remains the first choice for manufacturing the armours of the ITER divertor, even if the decrease of DBTT and the increase of ductility and fracture toughness are mandatory requirements for a successful application of the material. Aiming for this goal, three approaches are currently being studied to ductilize W [17,39,40]: (i) the preparation of W solid solutions (Re, Ir, Ta, and V are the most promising alloying elements), (ii) the synthesis of ultra-fine-grained W, and (iii) the synthesis of W composites. The last one consists in reinforcing a W matrix through W fibres coated by an engineered interface and seems to guarantee the best results.

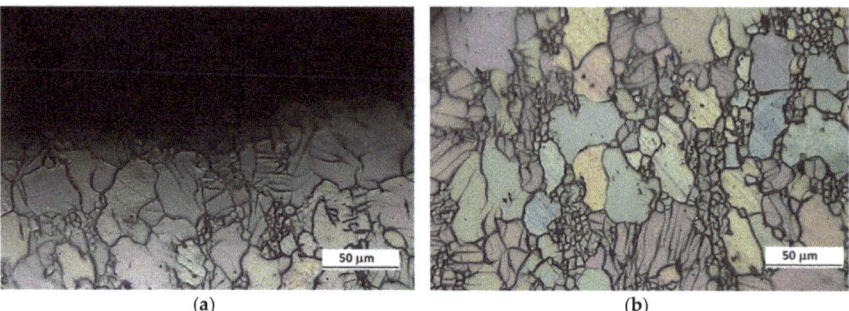

(a) (b)

Figure 10. (a) Cross-section of the crater and (b) of the zone just below.

4. Conclusions

The effects on Mo of transient high energy thermal loads occurring in a Tokamak during operative conditions have been simulated through a single laser pulse delivered by a Nd:YAG/Glass laser.

The examination of the irradiated zone evidenced that an erosion crater forms in the spot's central area due to metal vaporization and the ejection of molten metal. The thermal gradient leads to radial flushing of liquid metal, giving rise to a ridge around the crater and long filaments along the crater walls. Moreover, in a more external area (up to a distance of about 1 mm from the laser spot center), the surface shows bubbles and long cracks.

The results have been compared to those of previous experiments carried out in the same conditions on W, the material considered to be the principal candidate for building the armours of ITER.

Although some morphological features, namely the presence of an erosion crater at the centre of a more extended zone with surface modifications, are similar in Mo and W, these metals exhibit relevant differences:

- the crater is larger and shallower in the case of Mo;
- the volume of Mo ablated from the surface by a single laser pulse is about ten times that of W owing to the remarkably higher latent heat of fusion and latent heat of vaporization of W;
- the morphological features of the Mo crater walls are characterized by long filaments, not observed in the case of W, because the lower viscosity and surface tension of Mo allow an easier flow of the liquid metal;
- grain growth has been observed in a material layer of about 1 mm under the crater, with the effects decreasing as the distance from the surface increases.

In conclusion, the higher erosion of Mo indicates that W remains the best solution for manufacturing the armours of the ITER divertor.

Author Contributions: Conceptualization, R.M., E.P., R.R., M.R. and A.V.; Data curation, R.M., E.P., R.R., M.R. and A.V.; Investigation, E.P., R.R., M.R. and A.V.; Supervision, R.M.; Writing—original draft, R.M., E.P. and M.R. All authors have read and agreed to the published version of the manuscript.

Funding: This work has been carried out within the framework of the EUROfusion Consortium and has received funding from the Euratom research and training programme 2014–2018 and 2019–2020 under Grant Agreement No. 633053. The views and opinions expressed herein do not necessarily reflect those of the European Commission.

Acknowledgments: The authors are grateful to Piero Plini and Benedetto Iacovone of Department of Industrial Engineering for the assistance in sample preparation.

Conflicts of Interest: The authors declare no conflict of interest.

References

1. Riccardi, B.; Pizzuto, A.; Orsini, A.; Libera, S.; Visca, E.; Bertamini, L.; Casadei, F.; Severini, E.; Montanari, R.; Vesprini, R.; et al. Tungsten thick coatings for plasma facing components. *Fusion Technol.* **1998**, *31*, 223–226.
2. Roedig, M.; Kuehnlein, W.; Linke, J.; Merola, M.; Rigal, E.; Schedler, B.; Visca, E. Investigation of tungsten alloys as plasma facing materials for the ITER divertor. *Fusion Eng. Des.* **2002**, *61*, 135–140. [CrossRef]
3. Bolt, H.; Barabash, V.; Krauss, W.; Linke, J.; Neu, R.; Suzuki, S.; Nyoshida, N. Materials for the plasma facing components of fusion reactors. *J. Nucl. Mater.* **2004**, *329*, 66–73. [CrossRef]
4. Uytdenhouwen, I.; Decreton, M.; Hirai, T.; Linke, J.; Pintsuk, G.; Van Oost, G. Influence of recrystallization on thermal shock resistance of various tungsten grades. *J. Nucl. Mater.* **2007**, *363*, 1099–1103. [CrossRef]
5. Maier, H.; Hirai, T.; Rubel, M.; Neu, R.; Mertens, P.; Greuner, H.; Hopf, C.; Matthews, G.F.; Neubauer, O.; Piazza, G.; et al. Tungsten and beryllium armour development for the JET ITER-like wall project. *Nucl. Fusion* **2007**, *47*, 222. [CrossRef]
6. Herrmann, A.; Greuner, H.; Fuchs, J.C.; de Marné, P.; Neu, R.; ASDEX Upgrade Team. Experiences with tungsten coatings in high heat flux tests and under plasma load in ASDEX Upgrade. *Phys. Scr.* **2009**, *T138*, 014059. [CrossRef]
7. Cui, S.; Simmonds, M.; Qin, W.; Ren, F.; Tynan, G.R.; Doerner, R.P.; Chen, R. Thermal conductivity reduction of tungsten plasma facing material due to helium plasma irradiation in PISCES using the improved 3-omega method. *J. Nucl. Mater.* **2017**, *486*, 267–273. [CrossRef]
8. Kajita, S.; De Temmerman, G.; Morgan, T.; Van Eden, S.; de Kruif, T.; Ohno, N. Thermal response of nanostructured tungsten. *Nucl. Fusion* **2014**, *54*, 033005. [CrossRef]
9. Uytdenhouwen, I.; Massaut, V.; Linke, J.; Van Oost, G. Plasma wall interaction phenomena on tungsten armour materials for fusion applications. In Proceedings of the International Youth Nuclear Congress 2008, Interlaken, Switzerland, 20–26 September 2008.
10. Lemahieu, N.; Linke, J.; Pintsuk, G.; Van Oost, G.; Wirtz, M.; Zhou, Z. Performance of yttrium doped tungsten under "edge localized mode"-like loading conditions. *Phys. Scr.* **2014**, *T159*, 014035. [CrossRef]
11. Shirokova, V.; Laas, T.; Ainsaar, A.; Priimets, J.; Ugaste, U.; Väli, B.; Gribkov, V.A.; Maslyaev, S.A.; Demina, E.V.; Dubrovsky, A.D.; et al. Armor materials' behavior under repetitive dense plasma shots. *Phys. Scr.* **2014**, *T161*, 014045. [CrossRef]
12. De Temmerman, G.C.; Bystrov, K.E.; Zielinski, J.J.; Balden, M.; Matern, G.; Arnas, C.; Marot, L. Nanostructuring of molybdenum and tungsten surfaces by low-energy helium ions. *J. Vac. Sci. Technol. A Vac. Surf. Film.* **2012**, *30*, 41306. [CrossRef]
13. Tripathi, J.K.; Novakowski, T.J.; Hassanein, A. Tailoring molybdenum nanostructure evolution by low energy He^+ ion irradiation. *Appl. Surf. Sci.* **2015**, *353*, 1070–1081. [CrossRef]
14. Sinclair, G.; Tripathi, J.K.; Diwakar, P.K.; Hassanein, A. Structural response of transient heat loading on molybdenum surface exposed to low-energy helium ion irradiation. *Nucl. Fusion* **2016**, *56*, 36005. [CrossRef]
15. Brooks, J.N.; El-Guebaly, L.; Hassanein, A.; Sizyuk, T. Plasma-facing material alternatives to tungsten. *Nucl. Fusion* **2015**, *55*, 43002. [CrossRef]
16. Sinclair, G.; Tripathi, J.K.; Diwakar, P.K.; Hassanein, A. Melt layer erosion during ELM-like heat loading on molybdenum as an alternative plasma-facing material. *Sci. Rep.* **2017**, *7*, 12273. [CrossRef]
17. Rieth, M.; Dudarev, S.L.; De Vicente, S.M.G.; Aktaa, J.; Ahlgren, T.; Antusch, S.; Armstrong, D.E.J.; Balden, M.; Baluc, N.; Barthe, M.-F.; et al. Recent progress in research on tungsten materials for nuclear fusion applications in Europe. *J. Nucl. Mater.* **2013**, *432*, 482–500. [CrossRef]
18. Cottrell, G.A. Sigma phase formation in irradiated tungsten, tantalum and molybdenum in a fusion power plant. *J. Nucl. Mater.* **2004**, *334*, 166–168. [CrossRef]
19. Sizyuk, T.; Hassanein, A. Dynamic analysis and evolution of mixed materials bombarded with multiple ions beams. *J. Nucl. Mater.* **2010**, *404*, 60. [CrossRef]

20. Sharpe, J.P.; Kolasinski, R.D.; Shimada, M.; Calderoni, P.; Causey, R.A. Retention behavior in tungsten and molybdenum exposed to high fluences of deuterium ions in TPE. *J. Nucl. Mater.* **2009**, *390*, 709–712. [CrossRef]
21. Richetta, M.; Gaudio, P.; Montanari, R.; Pakhomova, E.; Antonelli, L. Laser pulse simulation of high energy transient thermal loads on bulk and plasma sprayed W for NFR. *Mater. Sci. Forum* **2017**, *879*, 1576–1581. [CrossRef]
22. Montanari, R.; Pakhomova, E.; Pizzoferrato, R.; Richetta, M.; Varone, A. Laser pulse effects on plasma sprayed and bulk tungsten. *Metals* **2017**, *7*, 454. [CrossRef]
23. Gaudio, P.; Montanari, R.; Pakhomova, E.; Richetta, M.; Varone, A. W-1%La$_2$O$_3$ submitted to a single laser pulse: Effect of particles on heat transfer and surface morphology. *Metals* **2018**, *8*, 389. [CrossRef]
24. Rubel, M.; Brezinsek, S.; Coenen, J.W.; Huber, A.; Kirschner, A.; Kreter, A.; Petersson, P.; Philipps, V.; Pospieszczyk, A.; Schweer, B.; et al. Overview of wall probes for erosion and deposition studies in the TEXTOR tokamak. *Matter Radiat. Extrem.* **2017**, *2*, 87–104. [CrossRef]
25. *International Centre for Diffraction Data*; JCPDS: Newtown Square, PA, USA, 1907.
26. Williamson, G.K.; Smallman, R.A. Dislocation densities in some annealed and cold-worked metals from measurements on the X-ray Debye-Scherrer spectrum. *Philos. Mag.* **1956**, *1*, 34–45. [CrossRef]
27. Gondi, P.; Donato, A.; Montanari, R.; Sili, A. Miniaturized test method for the mechanical characterization of structural materials for fusion reactors. *J. Nucl. Mater.* **1996**, *233*, 1557–1560. [CrossRef]
28. Francucci, M.; Gaudio, P.; Martellucci, S.; Richetta, M. Spectroscopy methods and applications of the Tor Vergata laser-plasma facility driven by GW-level laser system. *Int. J. Spectrosc.* **2011**, *2011*. [CrossRef]
29. Dong, H.; Wen, B.; Melnik, R. Relative importance of grain boundaries and size effects in thermal conductivity of nanocrystalline materials. *Nat. Sci. Rep.* **2014**, *4*, 7037. [CrossRef]
30. Swartz, E.T.; Pohl, R.O. Thermal boundary resistance. *Rev. Mod. Phys.* **1989**, *61*, 605. [CrossRef]
31. Nan, C.-W.; Birringer, R.; Clarke, D.R.; Gleiter, H. Effective thermal conductivity of particulate composites with interfacial thermal resistance. *J. Appl. Phys.* **1997**, *81*, 6692–6699. [CrossRef]
32. Yang, H.-S.; Bai, G.-R.; Thompson, L.; Eastman, J. Interfacial thermal resistance in nanocrystalline yttria-stabilized zirconia. *Acta Mater.* **2002**, *50*, 2309–2317. [CrossRef]
33. Paradis, P.F.; Ishikawa, T.; Koike, N. Non-contact measurements of the surface tension and viscosity of molybdenum using an electrostatic levitation furnace. *Int. J. Refract. Met. Hard Mater.* **2007**, *25*, 95–100. [CrossRef]
34. Paradis, P.F.; Ishikawa, T.; Fujii, R.; Yoda, S. Physical properties of liquid and undercooled tungsten by levitation techniques. *Appl. Phys. Lett.* **2005**, *86*, 041901. [CrossRef]
35. Cagran, C.; Wilthan, B.; Pottlacher, G. Normal spectral emissivity at a wavelength of 684.5 nm and thermophysical properties of solid and liquid molybdenum. In Proceedings of the 5th Symposium on Thermophysical Properties, Boulder, CO, USA, 23–28 June 2003.
36. Ishikawa, T.; Paradis, P.-F.; Okada, J.T.; Kumar, M.V.; Watanabe, Y. Viscosity of molten Mo, Ta, Os, Re, and W measured by electrostatic levitation. *J. Chem. Thermodyn.* **2013**, *65*, 1–6. [CrossRef]
37. Straus, J.; Kolacek, K.; Schmidt, J.; Frolov, O.; Vilemova, M.; Matejicek, J.; Jager, A.; Juha, L.; Toufarova, M.; Choukourov, A.; et al. Response of fusion plasma-facing materials to nanosecond pulses of extreme ultraviolet radiation. *Laser Part. Beam* **2018**, *36*, 293–307. [CrossRef]
38. Eksaeva, A.; Borodin, D.; Romazanov, J.; Kirschner, A.; Kreter, A.; Eichler, M.; Rasinski, M.; Pospieszczyk, A.; Unterberg, B.; Brezinsek, S.; et al. Surface roughness effect on Mo physical sputtering and re-deposition in the linear plasma device PSI-2 predicted by ERO2.0. *Nucl. Mater. Energy* **2019**, *19*, 13–18. [CrossRef]
39. Wurster, S.; Baluc, N.; Battabyal, M.; Crosby, T.; Du, J.; Garca-Rosales, C.; Hasegawa, A.; Hoffmann, A.; Kimura, A.; Kurishita, H.; et al. Recent progress in R&D on tungsten alloys for divertor structural and plasma facing materials. *J. Nucl. Mater.* **2013**, *442*, S181–S189.
40. Linsmeier, C.; Rieth, M.; Aktaa, J.; Chikada, T.; Hoffmann, A.; Hoffmann, J.; Houben, A.; Kurishita, H.; Jin, X.; Li, M.; et al. Development of advanced high heat flux and plasma-facing materials. *Nucl. Fusion* **2017**, *57*, 092007. [CrossRef]

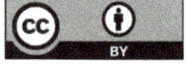

© 2020 by the authors. Licensee MDPI, Basel, Switzerland. This article is an open access article distributed under the terms and conditions of the Creative Commons Attribution (CC BY) license (http://creativecommons.org/licenses/by/4.0/).

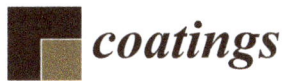

Article

Effect of 0.8 at.% H on the Mechanical Properties and Microstructure Evolution of a Ti–45Al–9Nb Alloy Under Uniaxial Tension at High Temperature

Qiqi Yu [1], Daosheng Wen [1,*], Shouren Wang [1,*], Beibei Kong [2], Shuxu Wu [1] and Teng Xiao [1]

1. School of Mechanical Engineering, University of Jinan, Jinan 250022, China; 20172120498@mail.ujn.edu.cn (Q.Y.); 20172120503@mail.ujn.edu.cn (S.W.); 201821200544@mail.ujn.edu.cn (T.X.)
2. Department of Mechanical Engineering, Shandong Jiaotong University, Jinan 250022, China; kongbeibei@sdjtu.edu.cn
* Correspondence: me_wends@ujn.edu.cn (D.W.); me_wangsr@ujn.edu.cn (S.W.)

Received: 8 November 2019; Accepted: 24 December 2019; Published: 7 January 2020

Abstract: To investigate the effect of hydrogen on the high-temperature deformation behaviors of TiAl-based alloys, the high-temperature tensile experiment was carried out on a Ti–45Al–9Nb (at.%) alloy with the H content of 0 and 0.8 at.%, respectively. Then, the effect of hydrogen on the high-temperature mechanical properties of the as-cast alloy was studied, the constitutive relations among stress, temperature, and strain rate were established, and the microstructure was analyzed. The results indicated that, compared with the unhydrogenated alloy, the flow stress of the hydrogenated alloy was significantly reduced, and the peak stress of the hydrogenated alloy decreased by $(16.28 \pm 0.17)\%$ deformed at $1150\ °C/0.0004\ s^{-1}$. Due to the presence of hydride $(TiAl)H_x$ in the alloy, the elongation showed a decline trend with increasing strain rate at the same deformation temperature. Compared with the unhydrogenated alloy, the elongation of the hydrogenated alloy reduced by $(26.05 \pm 0.45)\%$ $(0.0004\ s^{-1})$, $(23.49 \pm 0.38)\%$ $(0.001\ s^{-1})$, and $(14.23 \pm 0.19)\%$ $(0.0025\ s^{-1})$, respectively, indicating that 0.8 at.% H softened the Ti–45Al–9Nb alloy and reduced the high-temperature plastic deformability. Under the same deformation condition, the deformation extent of the hydrogenated alloy was less than that of the unhydrogenated alloy. There were more residual lamellae in the hydrogenated alloy, and the extent of dynamic recrystallization was lower than that of the unhydrogenated alloy.

Keywords: TiAl-based alloys; hydrogen-induced softening; dynamic recrystallization; cracking

---

1. Introduction

TiAl-based alloys are characterized by low density, high specific strength, excellent oxidation resistance, and creep resistance at high-temperature, so it is considered as one of the most promising high-temperature lightweight structural materials used in key components such as aerospace aircraft and automobile engines [1–3]. Due to the poor plasticity of TiAl-based alloys at room temperature, it is difficult to process and deform at room temperature. Furthermore, TiAl-based alloys have a high flow stress even in the thermal deformation process, so high performance dies and equipment are required in plastic forming [4,5]. Therefore, this requires that the dies and equipment can bear a higher load at temperatures of more than 1000 °C, and can work at a high-temperature for a long time, which virtually increases the cost and affects its practical process. Hence, these problems have become serious restrictions in the application of TiAl-based alloys.

In order to reduce the flow stress in the hot working process of TiAl-based alloys, researchers have mainly adopted an alloy composition design and microstructure control [6,7]. A large number of studies have proven that the addition of the alloying element Mo to TiAl-based alloys is an effective method to reduce the flow stress of TiAl-based alloys [8]. Godor et al. [9] studied the high-temperature deformation behavior of a high Mo–TiAl alloy, and found that the true stress–strain curve of the Ti–45Al–3Mo–0.5Si–0.1B alloy presented typical dynamic recrystallization softening characteristics. Based on the actual compression results, it was found that TiAl-based alloys had a relatively low flow stress and excellent thermal processing performance under the conditions of higher than 1100 °C and lower than 0.01 s^{-1}. However, the density of Mo is very large (i.e., 10.22 g/cm^3, almost twice as that of Ti), and Mo addition will greatly increases the density of the alloy. Therefore, a way needs to be found that can reduce the flow stress of TiAl-based alloys and does not increase the density. Thermohydrogen treatment (THT) (hydrogenation–hot working–vacuum dehydrogenation) takes hydrogen as a temporary alloying element. It reduces the flow stress of TiAl-based alloys without increasing density, and provides a new way to promote the practical application of TiAl-based alloys [10]. At present, Russia has successfully applied this technology in the production process of BT30 alloy bracket nuts and BT16 alloy large-diameter bolts [11]. Senkov et al. [12] studied the effect of hydrogen on the high-temperature mechanical behavior of a Ti–6Al–4V alloy and found that the peak stress of the alloy with a hydrogen content of 0.4 wt.% decreased by 70% when compared with the unhydrogenated one. Wen et al. [13] studied the influence of hydrogen on the high-temperature deformation behavior of the Ti–46Al–2V–1Cr–0.3Ni alloy and Ti–45Al–5Nb–0.8Mo–0.3Y alloy, and their maximum hydrogen absorption capability was 0.8 and 1.5 at.%, respectively. The results indicated that the peak stress of the Ti–46Al–2V–1Cr–0.3Ni alloy was reduced by 35% due to hydrogen addition when compressed at 1150 °C/0.01 s^{-1}. Under the compression deformation condition of 1200 °C and 0.01 s^{-1}, the peak stress of the Ti–45Al–5Nb–0.8Mo–0.3Y alloy was reduced by approximately 25% by hydrogen. Ma et al. [14] studied the effect of hydrogen on the high-temperature deformation behavior of the Ti–44Al–6Nb alloy and found that the alloy containing 0.2 wt.% hydrogen was compressed in a temperature range of 900–1000 °C, and its peak stress was decreased significantly, mainly because hydrogen promoted the dynamic recrystallization and spheroidization of the α_2 phase, increased the content of the β phase, and promoted the dynamic recovery of the β phase. Liu et al. [15] found that adding 0.3–0.5 at.% hydrogen in a Ti–47Al alloy could reduce the forging temperature of the alloy from 950 °C to 750 °C without increasing the deformation stress, which was of great significance to reduce mold wear, improve mold service life, and reduce cost.

Previous works have mainly focused on the effect of hydrogen on the mechanical properties and microstructure evolution of TiAl-based alloys under compressive stress. However, some microstructure characteristics and indices on hot workability cannot be observed and investigated under compressive stress, for example, elongation, which is one of the significant indices to reflect the hot workability. Up to now, systematic works on the effect of hydrogen on the hot workability of TiAl-based alloys under tensile stress have not been reported. Therefore, an isothermal tensile test was carried out to investigate the effect of hydrogen on the mechanical properties and microstructure evolution of a TiAl-based alloy in this paper.

2. Experiment

The nominal component of the TiAl-based alloy was Ti–45Al–9Nb (at.%). The original experimental material was an as-cast ingot with a diameter of 85 mm and a height of 89 mm. After casting, the ingot was hot isostatic pressed at 1260 °C for 4 h, with a gas pressure of 150 MPa, and then was soaked at 900 °C for 12 h. Finally, it was processed into the tensile specimens by wire cut electrical discharge machining (WEDM) and machining methods. Figure 1 shows the high-temperature tensile test specimen size of the Ti–45Al–9Nb alloy.

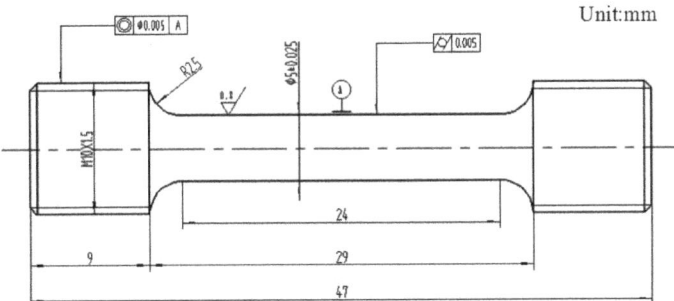

Figure 1. High-temperature tensile test specimen size of the Ti–45Al–9Nb alloy.

2.1. Hydrothermal Treatment

The tensile samples first underwent high-temperature hydrogenation. The specific process was as follows: first, the samples were placed in acetone for ultrasonic cleaning for 20 min, and then placed in a tube furnace; after vacuum up to 10^{-3} Pa, argon gas was filled; after the furnace temperature rose to 800 °C, the hydrogen was filled with an absolute pressure of 0.1–0.15 MPa, and then the samples were soaked for 2 h. When the furnace was cooled to room temperature, samples with H content of 0.8 at.% (abbreviated as 0.8 H below) were finally obtained. The highest hydrogen content obtained by the current hydrogenation equipment was only 0.8 at.%, which had the most significant effect on the mechanical properties and microstructure evolution of the present alloy, and so the study focused on a 0.8 at.% hydrogen. The hydrogen content was examined by a LECO-ROH600 oxygen/hydrogen analyzer (LECO, St Joseph, MI, USA), with an accuracy of 0.01 ppm. The error of the hydrogen content was ±3%. In order to accurately compare and study the effect of H on the high-temperature tensile deformation behavior and microstructure evolution of the Ti–45Al–9Nb alloy, the samples without hydrogen had a vacuum heat treatment with the same heat treatment system (without hydrogen addition).

2.2. High-Temperature Tensile Test

High-temperature uniaxial tensile test of the unhydrogenated and hydrogenated Ti–45Al–9Nb alloy samples was carried out on an MTS 880 universal tensile test machine by using the equivalent strain rate tensile method. The specific experimental process was as follows: first, the surface of the samples was sprayed with antioxidant alumina to prevent the surface oxidation; second, the samples were heated to the test temperature in a three-section circular resistance furnace, and had heat preservation for 10 min. The test temperatures were 1050, 1100, and 1150 °C and the strain rates were 0.0004, 0.001, and 0.0025 s^{-1}, respectively, and water-quenching was carried out immediately after the test. Finally, the stress–strain curves and deformed samples were obtained. The deformation behaviors of the alloy at the temperature of 1150 °C and the strain rate of 0.0004–0.0025 s^{-1} were mainly investigated in this paper.

2.3. Microstructural Analysis

The gauge part of samples after tensile deformation was wire-electrode cut, and then the surface to be observed was ground with 240, 400, and 600-grit SiC papers. Finally, electropolishing was carried out. The electrolytic polishing solution was 60% methanol + 34% n-butanol + 6% perchloric acid, the power supply voltage was adjusted to 20 V, the current maintained at 0.5–0.6 A, and the electrolysis time was 50 s.

Scanning electron microscopy (SEM) (JSM-7800F, Jeol, Tokyo, Japan) was used to analyze the microstructure of the gauge part of samples after high-temperature tension.

An X-ray diffractometer (XRD) (BRUKER Company, Karlsruhe, Germany, model: D8 ADVANCE) was used to analyze the phase. The radiation light used in the experiment was Cu Kα with a wavelength of 1.5418 Å, the generator's power was 1.6 kW (40 kV, 40 mA), the continuous scanning range was 10°–90°, the scanning rate was 0.2°/s, the step scanning step length was 0.02°, and each step lasted for one second.

3. Results and Discussion

3.1. Effect of Hydrogen on the Microstructure of Alloy at Room Temperature

SEM microstructures of the unhydrogenated and hydrogenated alloys are shown in Figure 2. Note that the dark gray phase is the γ phase, the light gray phase is the α_2 phase, and the bright white phase is the B2 phase. The α_2 phase is the ordered phase of the α phase at low temperature, and the B2 phase is the ordered phase of the β phase at low temperature. The microstructures of both alloys were near-lamellar, which were mainly composed of γ/α_2-lamellar colonies with an average size of about 800 µm. In addition, a small number of equiaxed γ grains and irregular B2 grains were distributed along the lamellar boundaries.

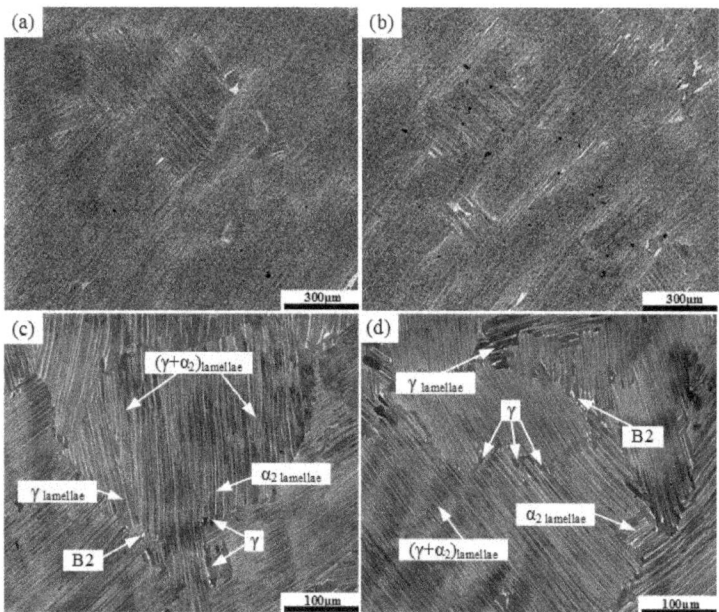

Figure 2. SEM microstructures of the unhydrogenated (**a,c**) and hydrogenated (**b,d**) Ti–45Al–9Nb alloys. (**c,d**) are the magnified images of (**a,b**), respectively.

Figure 3 shows the X-ray diffraction patterns of the unhydrogenated and hydrogenated Ti–45Al–9Nb alloys. Both the unhydrogenated and hydrogenated alloys were composed of a large amount of the γ phase ($L1_0$ crystal structure, $a = b = 0.4005$ nm, $c = 0.407$ nm, $a/c = 0.984$), a certain amount of the α_2 phase ($D0_{19}$ crystal structure, $a = b = 0.578$ nm, $c = 0.465$ nm, $a/c = 1.243$), and a very small amount of the B2 phase (CsCl crystal structure, $a = b = c = 0.316$ nm). The diffraction peaks of the α_2 phase, γ phase, and B2 phase were basically unchanged after hydrogen addition, and the intensity of the diffraction peaks of the α_2 phase and B2 phase was slightly stronger than that of the unhydrogenated alloy, indicating that hydrogen increased the content of the α_2 phase and B2 phase. In addition, the diffraction peak of the (TiAl)H_x hydride was found at 2θ = 35.46° after hydrogen addition. Meanwhile, the hydride had a tetragonal crystal structure with lattice constants $a = 0.452$ nm, $c = 0.326$ nm, and $c/a = 0.721$ [16]. The hydrogenation treatment of TiAl-based alloys was achieved by the diffusion of hydrogen atoms. In the diffusion process, hydrogen was first decomposed into hydrogen atoms and bumped into the surface of the samples. Due to a large number of defects and higher energy in the grain boundary or phase boundary, a channel was provided for the diffusion of hydrogen atoms. Therefore, hydrogen atoms preferentially diffused in a short range along the grain boundary or phase boundary, so the hydrogen concentration at the grain boundary or phase boundary reached saturation in a short time. Therefore, the concentration of hydrogen atoms at the grain boundary or phase boundary was relatively high, which could easily meet the requirements of composition fluctuation and energy fluctuation for hydride nucleation. When the hydrogen content exceeded its saturated solid solubility, the hydrogen combined with titanium aluminum to form titanium aluminum hydride.

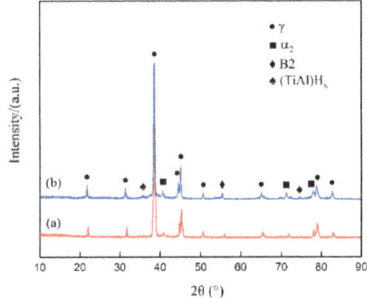

Figure 3. XRD patterns of the unhydrogenated (**a**) and hydrogenated (**b**) Ti–45Al–9Nb alloys.

In order to quantitatively study the content of each phase in the unhydrogenated and hydrogenated alloys, a quantitative XRD analysis was conducted. Figure 4 shows the relative volume fraction of the γ, α_2, B2, and (TiAl)H$_x$ phases in the unhydrogenated and hydrogenated alloys, which are calculated based on the integration area of the diffraction peaks. The contents of the γ, α_2, and B2 phases in the unhydrogenated alloy were 77.54%, 20.89%, and 1.57%, respectively, while the contents of the γ, α_2, and B2 phase in the hydrogenated alloy were 69.31%, 26.18%, and 2.85%, respectively. In general, hydrogen treatment can reduce the content of the γ phase because adding H can effectively promote the diffusion of elements and distort the γ phase lattice, thus promoting the $\gamma \rightarrow \alpha_2$ phase transformation [17]. In addition, the content of the B2 phase in the hydrogenated alloy was also slightly increased, indicating that hydrogen can stabilize the B2 phase and promote its precipitation.

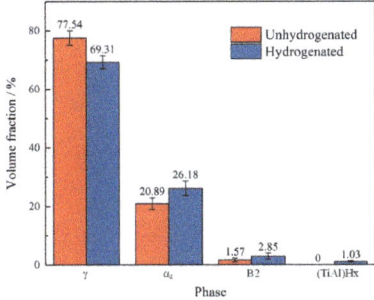

Figure 4. Volume fraction of phases in the unhydrogenated and hydrogenated Ti–45Al–9Nb alloys.

3.2. High-Temperature Flow Behavior of Hydrogenated Alloy

3.2.1. True Stress–True Strain Curves and Their Characteristics

Figure 5 shows the tensile deformed specimens and true stress–true strain curves of the unhydrogenated and hydrogenated Ti–45Al–9Nb alloys. Figure 5a shows the deformed specimens. Deformed at 1150 °C, all samples underwent a certain plastic deformation. Under the same deformation condition, the plastic deformation degree of the unhydrogenated alloy was greater than that of the hydrogenated alloy. Figure 5b–d show the true stress–true strain curves of the unhydrogenated and hydrogenated Ti–45Al–9Nb alloy samples deformed at 1150 °C, with strain rates of 0.0004, 0.001 and 0.0025 s^{-1}, respectively. Works have reported that if the stress dramatically drops after peak stress with increasing strain, the stress–strain curve is related to dynamic recrystallization [18]. Accordingly, the stress–strain curves shown in Figure 5b–d are supposed to be related to dynamic recrystallization. In the early stage of deformation, dislocation movement was gradually obstructed by increasing the dislocation propagation, resulting in a dislocation pileup, which increased the dislocation density and formed dislocation tangles. Meanwhile, a great stress concentration would be generated at the junction of lamellar colonies. This dislocation tangle and stress concentration would increase the flow stress and lead to work hardening, and macroscopically, the stress increased rapidly with the increase in strain until the stress reached its peak [19]. Subsequently, the stress decreased with an increase in the strain, which was mainly attributed to the increase of dynamic recrystallization. Dynamic recrystallization softening and the work hardening phase offset each other. When the softening effect of dynamic recrystallization was greater than the hardening effect of hot working, the strain tended to decrease significantly with the increase of the strain.

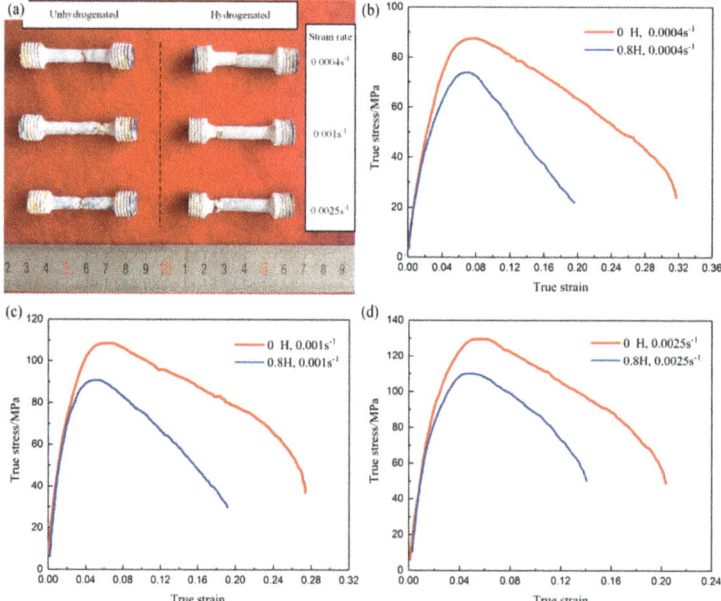

Figure 5. Tensile deformed specimens (**a**) and true stress-true strain curves (**b–d**) of the unhydrogenated and hydrogenated Ti–45Al–9Nb alloys deformed at (**b**) 1150 °C/0.0004 s^{-1}, (**c**) 1150 °C/0.001 s^{-1}, and (**d**) 1150 °C/0.0025 s^{-1}.

In addition, under the same deformation condition, the stress level of the hydrogenated alloy was lower than that of the unhydrogenated alloy, and the peak strain (the strain corresponded by the peak stress) of the hydrogenated alloy was lower than that of the unhydrogenated alloy. The smaller the peak strain, the sooner the dynamic recrystallization occurred [20]. The effects of hydrogen on the peak stress and elongation of the Ti–45Al–9Nb alloy at different strain rates are discussed in detail below.

3.2.2. Effect of Strain Rate on Flow Stress and Elongation

Figure 6 shows the peak stress and elongation of the unhydrogenated and hydrogenated Ti–45Al–9Nb alloys deformed in a strain rate range 0.0004–0.0025 s^{-1}, with a temperature of 1150 °C. As can be seen from Figure 6a,b, the peak stresses of the hydrogenated alloy and hydrogen decreased with the decrease in the strain rate, and the decrease trend tended to become flatter with the decrease in strain rate. At the same strain rate, the stress level of the hydrogenated alloy was lower than that of the unhydrogenated alloy, and the decrease rate of the peak stress increased with the decrease in the strain rate. Obviously, the addition of hydrogen caused flow softening, and the effect of hydrogen-induced softening was more obvious when the strain rate was lower. When deformed at 0.0004 s^{-1}, the decrease rate of the peak stress was more obvious, which was (16.28 ± 0.17)% lower than that of the unhydrogenated alloy. The softening mechanism of the hydrogenated alloy mainly includes dynamic recovery and dynamic recrystallization. In the plastic deformation of TiAl-based alloys, dislocation slip and climbing usually occur [21]. When the deformation temperature is constant, dislocation glide and climb gain more time with the decrease in strain rate, which allows the dynamic recrystallization nucleation to take place more easily to some extent. Therefore, the peak stress of both the hydrogenated and hydrogenated alloys decreased with the decrease in strain rate.

In addition, from the perspective of dislocation velocity and critical shear stress, the increase in strain rate would increase the dislocation movement and further increase the critical shear stress of the dislocation movement. Their relationship can be expressed as follows [22]:

$$v = v_0 e^{(\frac{C}{T\tau})} \tag{1}$$

where v is the velocity dislocation movement; v_0 is the sound's propagation speed in titanium aluminum alloy; C is the material constant; T is the absolute temperature; and τ is the critical shear stress of dislocation movement.

According to Equation (1), under the condition of constant deformation temperature, the increase of v inevitably leads to the increase of τ, that is, the flow stress increases.

Figure 6c,d show the reduction rate of the elongation of the hydrogenated alloy when the temperature was 1150 °C and the strain rate was 0.0004–0.0025 s^{-1}. As can be seen from Figure 6c,d, the elongation of the alloy decreased with the increase in the strain rate. At the same deformation temperature, the elongation of the hydrogenated alloy was lower than that of the unhydrogenated alloy, which decreased by (26.05 ± 0.45)% (0.0004 s^{-1}), (23.49 ± 0.38)% (0.001 s^{-1}), and (14.23 ± 0.19)% (0.0025 s^{-1}), respectively, indicating that 0.8 at.% H reduced the high-temperature plasticity of Ti–45Al–9Nb under this deformation condition. This might be due to the fact that, in the hydrogenated alloy, hydrogen did not always exist in the alloy in the form of a solid solution, and that some hydrogen combined with alloy atoms to form hydride (TiAl)H$_x$. The results indicated that the hydride itself was a brittle phase, and that it could easily become a crack source and promote the generation of cracks [23,24]. Therefore, the plasticity of the hydrogenated alloy was reduced due to the existence of hydride (TiAl)H$_x$. In addition, as shown in Figure 6d, the reduction rate of hydrogenated elongation became smaller and smaller with the increase in the strain rate. This was mainly because with the increase in strain rate, the deformation time of the unhydrogenated alloy became shorter and shorter, and the dynamic recrystallization grain nucleation and growth were less likely to take place. Meanwhile, when the layer of lamellar colonies inside the plastic deformation was small, the pressure under the action of relative rotation took place between lamellar colonies, which easily caused the stress concentration in the process of the rotation of the lamellar colonies, resulting in too early deformation and instability of the alloy. Therefore, the hydrogenated alloy showed a significant reduction trend of elongation in the macroscopic view.

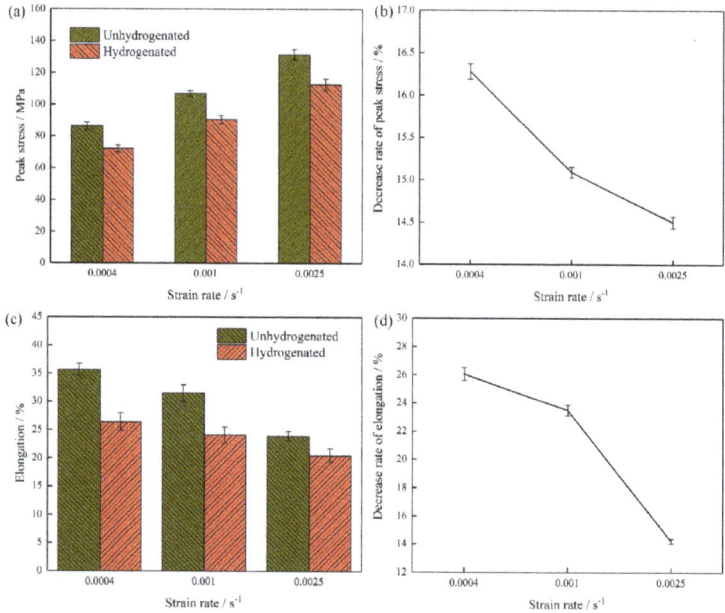

Figure 6. Peak stress and elongation of the unhydrogenated and hydrogenated Ti–45Al–9Nb alloys deformed in a strain rate range of 0.0004–0.0025 s^{-1}, with a temperature of 1150 °C. (**a**) Peak stresses and (**b**) the decrease rate of peak stress due to hydrogen addition, (**c**) elongation, and (**d**) the decrease rate of elongation due to hydrogen addition.

3.2.3. Constitutive Equation at High Temperature

A large number of works have indicated that the high-temperature deformation process of metal materials such as steel and iron materials, aluminum alloy, titanium alloy and TiAl-based alloy is through the thermal activation process. High-temperature flow behavior is controlled by deformation temperature and strain rate, and there is a constitutive relationship between flow stress σ, deformation temperature T, and strain rate $\dot{\varepsilon}$ (i.e., hyperbolic sine function), as shown in Equation (2) [25,26]:

$$\dot{\varepsilon} = A[\sinh(\alpha\sigma)]^n \exp\left(-\frac{Q}{RT}\right) \quad (2)$$

The relationship among σ, $\dot{\varepsilon}$, and T at a low stress (ασ < 0.8) is expressed as an exponential function:

$$\dot{\varepsilon} = A_1 \sigma^n \exp\left(-\frac{Q}{RT}\right) \quad (3)$$

The relationship among σ, $\dot{\varepsilon}$, and T at a high stress (ασ > 0.8) is expressed as an exponential function:

$$\dot{\varepsilon} = A_2 [\exp(\beta\sigma)] \exp\left(-\frac{Q}{RT}\right) \quad (4)$$

where n and n_1 are stress exponents, A, A_1, A_2; α and β are the material constants, among which α, β, and n_1 satisfies the relationship α = β/n_1; R is the gas constant; Q is the thermal deformation activation energy (KJ/mol); and T is the absolute temperature (K).

Assuming that deformation activation energy Q is independent of the deformation temperature T, and natural logarithms of both sides of the above three equations can be obtained as follows:

$$\ln \dot{\varepsilon} + \frac{Q}{RT} = \ln A + n\ln[\sinh(\alpha\sigma)] \qquad (5)$$

$$\ln \dot{\varepsilon} + \frac{Q}{RT} = \ln A_1 + n_1 \ln \sigma \qquad (6)$$

$$\ln \dot{\varepsilon} + \frac{Q}{RT} = \ln A_2 + \beta \sigma \qquad (7)$$

The partial derivatives of both sides of Equations (2)–(4) were obtained, and then n_1, β, and n can be expressed as follows:

$$n = \frac{\partial(\ln \dot{\varepsilon})}{\partial\{\ln[\sinh(\alpha\sigma)]\}}\bigg|_{1/T} \qquad (8)$$

$$n_1 = \frac{\partial(\ln \dot{\varepsilon})}{\partial(\ln \sigma)}\bigg|_{1/T} \qquad (9)$$

$$\beta = \frac{\partial(\ln \dot{\varepsilon})}{\partial \sigma}\bigg|_{1/T} \qquad (10)$$

The partial derivatives of both sides of Equations (5)–(7) were obtained, and then substituted into Equations (8)–(10) to calculate the expressions of n_1, β, and n, and the activation energy Q can be calculated.

All stress conditions:

$$Q = R\frac{\partial(\ln \dot{\varepsilon})}{\partial\{\ln[\sinh(\alpha\sigma)]\}}\bigg|_{1/T} \cdot \left\{\frac{\partial\{\ln[\sinh(\alpha\sigma)]\}}{\partial(1/T)}\right\}\bigg|_{\dot{\varepsilon}} \qquad (11)$$

Low stress:

$$Q = R\frac{\partial(\ln \dot{\varepsilon})}{\partial(\ln \sigma)}\bigg|_{1/T} \cdot \frac{\partial(\ln \sigma)}{\partial[\ln(1/T)]}\bigg|_{\dot{\varepsilon}} \qquad (12)$$

High stress:

$$Q = R\frac{\partial(\ln \dot{\varepsilon})}{\partial(\ln \sigma)}\bigg|_{1/T} \cdot \left\{\frac{\partial \sigma}{\partial[\ln(1/T)]}\right\}\bigg|_{\dot{\varepsilon}} \qquad (13)$$

The hyperbolic sine function (see Equation (2)) is more suitable to express the relationship between the peak stress and strain rate of the unhydrogenated and hydrogenated TiAl-based alloys [27]. According to the above-mentioned equations and experimental data, the relationships between the peak stress and strain rate of the unhydrogenated and hydrogenated Ti–45Al–9Nb alloys can be built. Figure 7 shows the relationships between σ_p and $\dot{\varepsilon}$ of the unhydrogenated and hydrogenated alloys. According to the curve fitting results, unary linear regression was carried out, the constant n_1 and β of the hydrogenated and unhydrogenated alloys could be obtained, where their n_1 were 4.55 ± 0.17 and 4.17 ± 0.13, respectively, and their β were 0.04 ± 0.02 and 0.05 ± 0.02, respectively. Later, the value of the α of the hydrogenated and unhydrogenated alloys can be calculated by the equation $\alpha = \beta/n_1$ as 0.009 ± 0.001 and 0.011 ± 0.001, respectively.

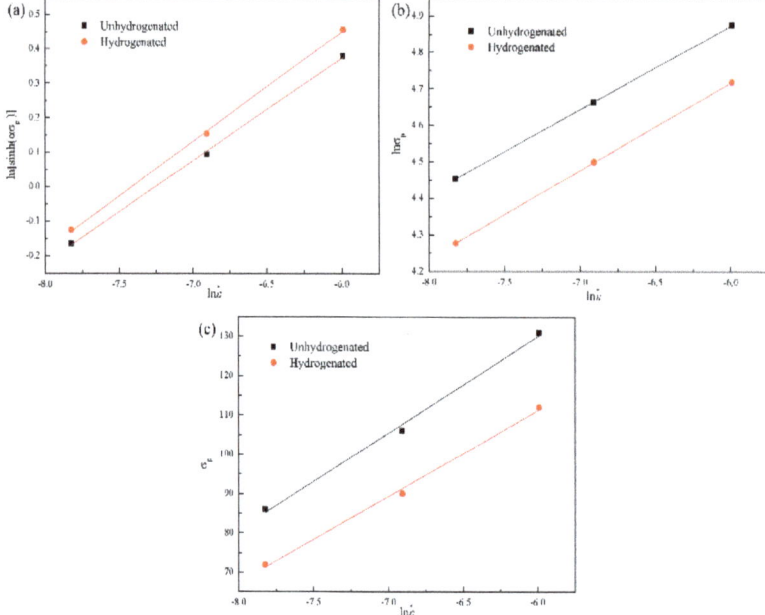

Figure 7. Relationships between σ_p and $\dot{\varepsilon}$ of the unhydrogenated and hydrogenated alloys: (a) $\ln[\sinh(\alpha\sigma_p)]$–$\ln \dot{\varepsilon}$; (b) $\ln\sigma_p$–$\ln \dot{\varepsilon}$ and (c) σ_p–$\ln \dot{\varepsilon}$ relationships.

α can be used to obtain the relation curve of $\ln \dot{\varepsilon}$–$\ln[\sinh(\alpha\sigma_p)]$, as shown in Figure 7c. According to Equation (8), the value of n can be calculated. The n values of the hydrogenated and unhydrogenated alloys were 3.37 ± 0.12 and 3.15 ± 0.11, respectively. Finally, the deformation activation energy Q can be calculated from the relationship between temperature T and strain rate $\dot{\varepsilon}$ of the unhydrogenated and hydrogenated alloys, as shown in Table 1. The Q values of the hydrogenated and unhydrogenated alloys were (584.31 ± 5.34) KJ/mol and (556.95 ± 4.15) KJ/mol, respectively.

Table 1. Constitutive equation parameter values of the hydrogenated and unhydrogenated alloys.

Samples	lnA	n	α	Q (KJ/mol)
Unhydrogenated	42.31 ± 0.83	3.37 ± 0.12	0.009 ± 0.001	584.31 ± 5.34
Hydrogenated	39.97 ± 0.69	3.15 ± 0.11	0.011 ± 0.001	556.95 ± 4.15

The constitutive equations of the Ti–45Al–9Nb alloy deformed at high-temperature can be obtained as follows:

Unhydrogenated:

$$\dot{\varepsilon} = e^{42.31}[\sinh(0.009\sigma)]^{3.37}\exp\left(-\frac{584310}{RT}\right) \tag{14}$$

Hydrogenated:

$$\dot{\varepsilon} = e^{39.97}[\sinh(0.011\sigma)]^{3.15}\exp\left(-\frac{556950}{RT}\right) \tag{15}$$

The above analysis indicates that for the Ti–45Al–9Nb alloy, the stress and deformation condition satisfied a hyperbolic sinusoidal relationship at high-temperature, and the deformation activation energy was significantly higher than the energy required for self-diffusion (290–345 KJ/mol) [28]. Therefore, the main softening mechanism for the unhydrogenated and hydrogenated alloys was dynamic recrystallization. Hydrogen decreased the deformation activation energy, which was mainly attributed to the fact that hydrogen could reduce the diffusion barrier, increase the diffusion coefficient of atoms, and coordinate deformation during thermal deformation. At the same time, hydrogen could promote dislocation movement, which led to a decrease in the thermal deformation activation energy.

3.3. Microstructure Evolution

Figure 8 shows the SEM images of the unhydrogenated and hydrogenated alloys deformed at 1150 °C and in the strain rate range of 0.0004–0025 s^{-1}. With the decrease in the strain rate, the deformation and the extent of dynamic recrystallization increased gradually. This is because the alloying element diffused sufficiently at a lower strain rate, which facilitated the decomposition of α_2 and γ phase lamellae. Therefore, the dynamic recrystallization took place more sufficiently. The decomposition of lamellae can also be regarded as a special dynamic recrystallization (DRX) process. It also includes nucleation (lamellar fragmentation) and growth (lamellar spheroidization) [29]. When the strain rate was 0.0025 s^{-1}, some lamellar colonies of the unhydrogenated and hydrogenated alloys were bent to a certain extent, showing a wavy shape. The orientation of the bent and deformed α_2/γ lamellar was a medium orientation, that is, the lamellar direction was perpendicular to the tensile direction. A small amount of block-shaped α_2 phase was formed at the grain boundary of the lamellar colonies in the unhydrogenated alloy. However, the hydrogenated alloy had fractured when the deformation was very small, thus it was difficult to observe the fracture or dynamic recrystallization structure. When the strain rate decreased to 0.001 s^{-1}, there were not only bending lamellar, but also a certain amount of lamellar fragmentation and spheroidized structures as well as fine dynamic recrystallization grains in the unhydrogenated alloy. It can be seen from Figure 8b,e that some lamellar colonies in the unhydrogenated alloy increased in spacing along the direction of stress, that is, the lamellar was obviously coarsened and accompanied by lamellar bending. The γ phase recrystallization grains occurred in the α_2/γ lamellar interface. As the number of α_2-phase slip systems was less than that of the γ phase, uncoordinated deformation and stress concentration easily occurred in the lamellar interface, which caused the lamellar interface to have local small deformation and provided driving energy for the recrystallization nucleation [30]. However, only a few lamellae were coarsened and the recrystallization grains were relatively less. When the strain rate dropped to 0.0004 s^{-1}, there were many bent and elongated lamellae. The spacing of the lamellar colonies was larger, the fragmentation of the lamellar colonies was enhanced, and the number and size of the recrystallization grains at the interface of the lamellar colonies increased obviously. In comparison, there were more residual lamellae and the extent of recrystallization was lower than that of the unhydrogenated alloy. According to the above analysis, dynamic recrystallization was very sensitive to the strain rate, and the smaller the strain rate, the more obvious the dynamic recrystallization. Under the same deformation condition, the deformation extent of the hydrogenated alloy was less than that of the unhydrogenated alloy, which was consistent with the elongation decrease in the hydrogenated alloy above-mentioned.

Through a comparison with previous work, it was found that the influence of hydrogen on the mechanical properties of the alloy was different during the high-temperature plastic deformation of the hydrogenated TiAl alloys. When the specimen was subject to tensile stress, hydrogen deteriorated the elongation of the Ti–45Al–9Nb alloy at high temperature. The main reason is that there are two forms of hydrogen in the alloys. On one hand, hydrogen atoms are dissolved in the lattice interstices. On the other hand, hydrogen atoms combine with alloy atoms to form hydride (i.e., $(TiAl)H_x$). After hydrogen entered the lattice sites, it weakens the binding force between the Ti and Al atoms, and reduces the binding energy [31]. The aggregation of hydrogen atoms along the grain boundary or phase boundary decreases the driving force for dislocation emission and movement, which leads to local plastic deformation and reduces the toughness. Meanwhile, the hydride gathers along the grain boundary, which is a source of cracking. The tensile stress accelerates the emergence and propagation of the grain boundary cracks, and finally results in deformation instability. Therefore, the elongation of the hydrogenated alloy was less than that of the unhydrogenated alloy. For most hydrogenated TiAl alloys using the solid hydrogenation technique, there is no hydride when compressive tests are conducted at high temperature [13–15]. When such hydrogenated specimens are compressed at high temperature, hydrogen can improve the plastic deformability, which is mainly due to hydrogen-induced dislocation movement, hydrogen-promoted dynamic recrystallization and twinning, and hydrogen-increased β phase content.

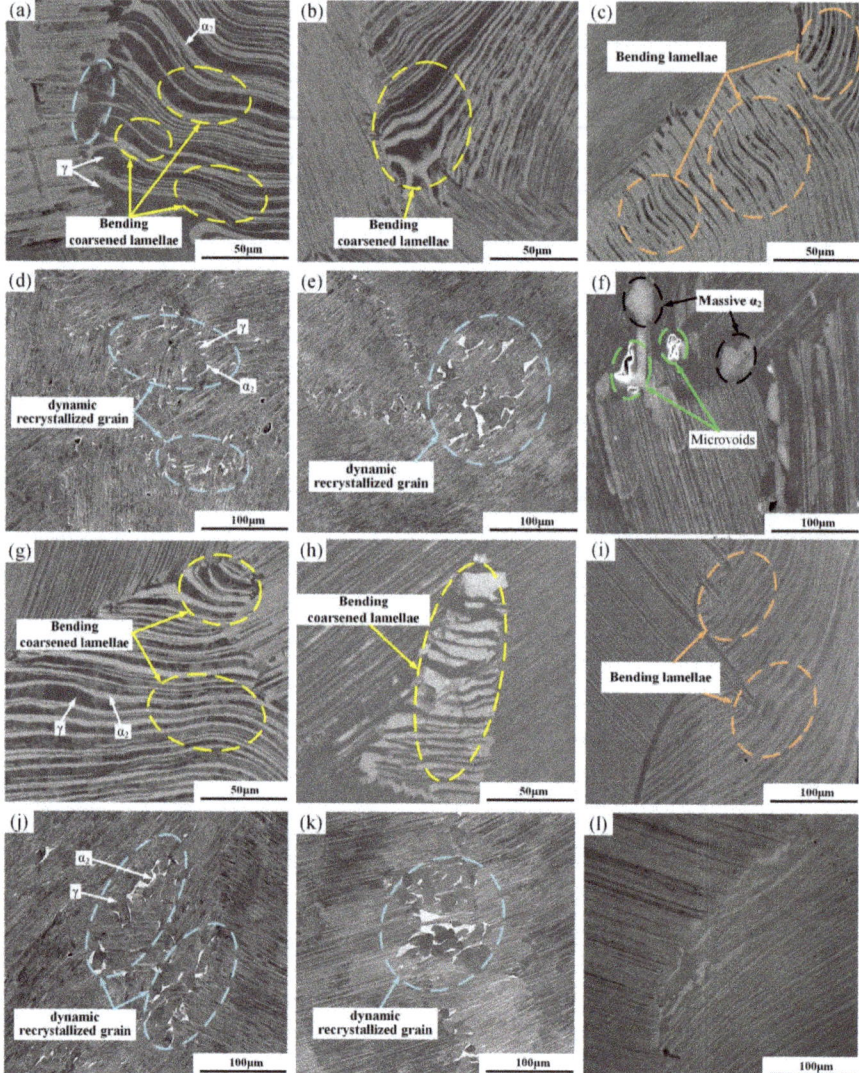

Figure 8. SEM images of the unhydrogenated (**a–f**) and hydrogenated (**g–l**) alloys deformed at (**a,d,g,j**) 1150 °C/0.0004 s^{-1}, (**b,e,h,k**) 1150 °C/0.001 s^{-1}, and (**c,f,i,l**) 1150 °C/0.0025 s^{-1}.

In order to study the mechanism of crack generation and propagation in hydrogen-containing alloys, we observed the cracks generated by the alloy under different deformation conditions and found that the internal crack propagation mechanism of the alloy was similar under this test condition. Therefore, crack generation and propagation under the deformation condition of 1150 °C/0.001 s^{-1} was chosen as the main research object. Figure 9 shows the cracking modes of the hydrogenated alloy deformed at 1150 °C/0.001 s^{-1}. The cracks mainly occurred in the internal lamellar colonies or at the boundary of the lamellar colonies. Among them, the internal cracks in the lamellar colonies were mainly generated at the α_2/γ lamellar boundary, which could be divided into inter-lamellar and trans-lamellar cracks, according to the different propagation techniques of cracks. These two kinds of cracks were mostly wedge cracks, which were mainly generated at the α_2/γ lamellar boundary and were caused by the deformation disharmony between the α_2 and γ lamellae. After crack nucleation was completed along the flat α_2/γ lamellar boundary, the crack continued to propagate along the α_2/γ lamellar boundary until reaching the lamellar colony boundaries, as shown in Figure 9a. Trans-lamellar cracks nucleated in the crooked α_2/γ lamellar boundary, and the crooked α_2/γ phase boundary retarded the propagation of cracks to some extent. These types of cracks were usually accompanied by bridging structures, as shown in Figure 9b. The cracks along the lamellar colony boundary were mainly generated in the α_2/γ lamellar colony boundary or the γ/γ lamellar colony boundary. Such cracks in the hydrogenated alloy were more than that in the unhydrogenated alloy. The accumulation of solid dissolved hydrogen and precipitated hydride at the grain boundary caused the stress concentration at the grain boundary, reduced the binding force at the boundary, and weakened lamellar colony boundaries, thus leading to more along-lamellar colony boundary cracks [32], as shown in Figure 9c. The propagation of such cracks was different from that of the inter-lamellar cracks. The along-lamellar colony boundary cracks formed a cavity after completing nucleation. Due to the occurrence of deformation in the alloy, crystal defects such as vacancies continuously increased, and in order to reduce the surface energy, these vacancies gathered along a certain direction under external stress, which made the cavity gradually grow and form a series of "cavity beads" along the lamellar colony boundaries. The cavities mutually combined to complete the crack propagation. The crack shown in Figure 9d is a combination of the above three types of cracks. Figure 10 is a schematic diagram of inter-lamellar, trans-lamellar, and along-lamellar colony boundary cracking propagation of the hydrogenated alloy.

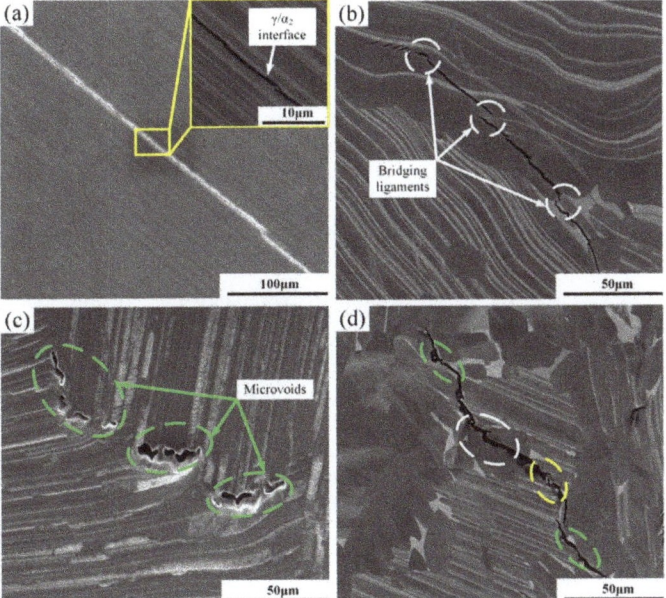

Figure 9. Cracking modes of the hydrogenated alloy deformed at 1150 °C/0.001 s^{-1}: (**a**) inter-lamellar crack, (**b**) trans-lamellar crack, (**c**) along-lamellar colony boundary crack, and (**d**) mixed mode crack.

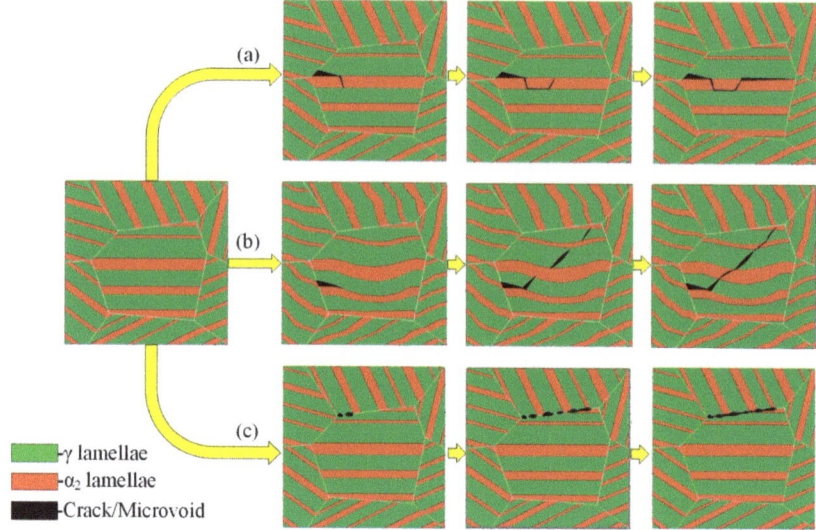

Figure 10. Schematic diagram of inter-lamellar (**a**), trans-lamellar (**b**), and along-lamellar colony boundary (**c**) cracking propagation of the hydrogenated alloy.

4. Conclusions

- Through hydrogen treatment, the phase content of the α_2 and B2 phases in the hydrogenated alloy increased when compared with that of the unhydrogenated alloy. In the hydrogenated alloy, hydride $(TiAl)H_x$ was observed, which led to cracks.
- Compared with the unhydrogenated alloy, the flow stress of the hydrogen alloy was significantly reduced (i.e., hydrogen-induced softening). Hydrogen-induced softening was enhanced with a decrease in the strain rate. Deformed at 1150 °C/0.0004 s^{-1}, the peak stress was decreased by (16.28 ± 0.17)% due to hydrogen addition. The elongation of the hydrogenated alloys was decreased by (26.05 ± 0.45)% (0.0004 s^{-1}), (23.49 ± 0.38)% (0.001 s^{-1}), and (14.23 ± 0.19)% (0.0025 s^{-1}), indicating that the addition of 0.8 at.% H reduced the high-temperature plasticity of Ti–45Al–9Nb alloy. In addition, the deformation activation energy of the hydrogenated alloy was lower than that of the unhydrogenated alloy.
- Under the same deformation condition, the deformation extent of the hydrogenated alloy was less than that of the unhydrogenated alloy. Accordingly, more residual lamellae and the lower extent of recrystallization were observed in the hydrogenated alloy. In addition, there were three types of cracks in the hydrogenated alloy (i.e., inter-lamellar, trans-lamellar, and along-lamellar colony boundary cracks). Furthermore, more along-lamellar colony boundary cracks occurred in the hydrogenated alloy.

Author Contributions: S.W. (Shouren Wang) and D.W. developed the experimental plan. Q.Y. wrote the main part of the manuscript. Q.Y. and S.W. (Shuxu Wu) tested the high temperature tensile properties of the different alloys and established the constitutive equation. Q.Y. and B.K. performed the characterization of the microstructure of the samples. Q.Y. and T.X. conducted the final typesetting of the article. S.W. (Shouren Wang) and D.W. summed up the article and conducted a final review. All authors have read and agreed to the published version of the manuscript.

Funding: This research was funded by the National Natural Science Foundation of China (51705199 and 51872122), the Natural Science Foundation of Shandong Province (ZR2017BEE055), the Key Technology Research and Development Program of Shandong (2019GGX104045 and 2017GGX30143), the Program for PhD Research Start-up Fund of Shandong Jiaotong University (Z201709), and the Taishan Scholar Engineering Special Funding (ts201511040).

Acknowledgments: We sincerely appreciate the support on the microstructure observation and analysis from the Analysis and Testing Center of Shandong University.

Conflicts of Interest: The authors declare no conflict of interest.

References

1. Liss, K.D.; Bartels, A.; Clemens, H.; Bystrzanowski, S.; Stark, A.; Buslaps, T.; Schimansky, F.P.; Gerling, R.; Scheu, C.; Schreyer, A. Recrystallization and phase transitions in a on TiAl-based alloy as observed by ex situ and in situ high-energy X-ray diffraction. *Acta Mater.* **2006**, *54*, 3721–3735. [CrossRef]
2. Kastenhuber, M.; Rashkova, B.; Clemens, H.; Mayer, S. Enhancement of creep properties and microstructural stability of intermetallic β-solidifying γ-TiAl based alloys. *Intermetallics* **2015**, *63*, 19–26. [CrossRef]
3. Zong, Y.Y.; Wen, D.S.; Guo, B.; Shan, D.B. Investigations of hydrogen-promoted $α_2$-lamella decomposition of a γ-TiAl based alloy. *Mater. Lett.* **2015**, *152*, 196–199. [CrossRef]
4. Wang, Q.; Ding, H.; Zhang, H.; Chen, R.; Guo, J.; Fu, H. Influence of Mn addition on the microstructure and mechanical properties of a directionally solidified γ-TiAl alloy. *Mater. Charact.* **2018**, *137*, 133–141. [CrossRef]
5. Zhang, C.P.; Zhang, K.F.; Wang, G.F. Dependence of heating rate in PCAS on microstructures and high-temperature deformation properties of γ-TiAl intermetallic alloys. *Intermetallics* **2010**, *18*, 834–840. [CrossRef]
6. Erdely, P.; Staron, P.; Maawad, E.; Schell, N.; Klose, J.; Mayer, S.; Clemens, H. Effect of hot rolling and primary annealing on the microstructure and texture of a β-stabilised γ-TiAl based alloy. *Acta Mater.* **2017**, *126*, 145–153. [CrossRef]
7. Huang, Z.W.; Lin, J.P.; Sun, H.L. Microstructural changes and mechanical behaviour of a near lamellar γ-TiAl alloy during long-term exposure at 700 °C. *Intermetallics* **2017**, *85*, 59–68. [CrossRef]
8. Hu, H.; Wu, X.Z.; Wang, R.; Li, W.G.; Liu, Q. Phase stability, mechanical properties and electronic structure of TiAl alloying with W, Mo, Sc and Yb: First-principles study. *J. Alloys Compd.* **2016**, *658*, 689–696. [CrossRef]
9. Godor, F.; Werner, R.; Lindemann, J.; Clemens, H.; Mayer, S. Characterization of the high-temperature deformation behavior of two intermetallic TiAl–Mo alloys. *Mater. Sci. Eng. A* **2015**, *648*, 208–216. [CrossRef]
10. Hou, H.L.; Li, Z.Q.; Wang, Y.J.; Guan, Q. Technology of hydrogen treatment for titanium alloy and its application prospect. *Chin. J. Nonferrous Met.* **2003**, *1*, 533–549.
11. Wang, J.W.; Gong, H.R. Adsorption and diffusion of hydrogen on Ti, Al, and TiAl surfaces. *Int. J. Hydrogen Energy* **2014**, *39*, 6068–6075. [CrossRef]
12. Senkov, O.N.; Jonas, J.J.; Froes, F.H. Thermally activated flow of β-titanium and β-titaniumhydrogen alloys. *Philos. Mag. A* **2000**, *80*, 2813–2825. [CrossRef]
13. Wen, D.S.; Huang, S.H.; Guo, B.; Shan, D.B.; Zong, Y.Y. Effect of hydrogen on γ-phase transformation and texture evolution of a TiAl-based alloy deformed at elevated temperature. *Mater. Sci. Eng. A* **2017**, *699*, 176–184. [CrossRef]
14. Ma, T.F.; Chen, R.R.; Zheng, D.S.; Liu, C. Hydrogenation behavior of Ti–44Al–6Nb alloy and its effect on the microstructure and hot deformability. *J. Mater. Res.* **2017**, *32*, 1304–1315. [CrossRef]
15. Liu, X.W.; Su, Y.Q.; Luo, L.S.; Li, K.; Dong, F.Y.; Guo, J.J.; Fu, H.Z. Effect of hydrogen treatment on solidification structures and mechanical properties of TiAl alloys. *Int. J. Hydrogen Energy* **2011**, *36*, 3260–3267. [CrossRef]
16. Chen, Y.L.; Zhang, T.; Song, L. Hydride formation during cathodic charging and its effect on mechanical properties of a high Nb containing TiAl alloy. *Int. J. Hydrogen Energy* **2018**, *43*, 8161–8169. [CrossRef]
17. Lei, J.; Fan, L. Effects of Hydrogen on Diffusion Bonding of TiAl-Based Intermetallics with Hydrogenated Ti6Al4V Alloy Interlayer Containing 0.5 wt.% Hydrogen. *Adv. Mater. Res.* **2013**, *750*, 624–629.
18. Xu, Y.S.; Liu, J.T.; Nie, M.; Li, Z.G.; Ruan, X.Y. Research and application of mathematical model for hot forming stress-strain curve. *J. Appl. Sci.* **1997**, *15*, 379–384.
19. Brotzu, A.; Felli, F.; Marra, F.; Pilone, D.; Pulci, G. Mechanical properties of a TiAl-based alloy at room and high-temperatures. *Mater. Sci. Technol.* **2018**, *34*, 1847–1853. [CrossRef]
20. He, X.M.; Yu, Z.Q.; Lai, X.M. Analysis of high-temperature deformation behavior of a high Nb containing TiAl based alloy. *Mater. Lett.* **2008**, *62*, 4181–4183. [CrossRef]
21. Liu, N.; Li, Z.; Xu, W.Y.; Wang, Y.; Zhang, G.Q.; Yuan, H. Hot deformation behavior and microstructural evolution of powder metallurgical TiAl alloy. *Rare Met.* **2016**, *36*, 236–241. [CrossRef]

22. Acharya, A.; Zhang, X.H. From dislocation motion to an additive velocity gradient decomposition, and some simple models of dislocation dynamics. *Chin. Ann. Math. B* **2015**, *36*, 645–658. [CrossRef]
23. Lunarska, E.; Chernyaeva, O.; Lisovytskii, D. Hydride formation under cathodic charging of titanium and TiAl-based alloys in alkaline solutions. *Mater. Sci.* **2008**, *44*, 423–428. [CrossRef]
24. Kazantseva, N.V.; Popov, A.G.; Mushnikov, N.V.; Soloninin, A.V.; Aleksashin, B.A.; Novozhenov, V.I.; Sazonova, V.A.; Kharisova, A.G. Thermally unstable hydrides of titanium aluminide Ti$_3$Al. *Phys. Met. Metallogr.* **2011**, *111*, 353–360. [CrossRef]
25. Li, T.R.; Liu, G.H.; Xu, M.; Niu, H.Z.; Fu, T.L.; Wang, Z.D.; Wang, G.D. Microstructures and high-temperature Tensile Properties of Ti-43Al-4Nb-1.5Mo Alloy in the canned forging and heat treatment process. *Acta Meter. Sin.* **2017**, *53*, 1055–1064.
26. Ding, J.; Lin, J.P.; Zhang, M.; Dong, C.L.; Liang, Y.F. High-temperature torsion induced gradient microstructures in high Nb-TiAl alloy. *Mater. Lett.* **2017**, *209*, 193–196. [CrossRef]
27. Narayana, P.L.; Li, C.L.; Hong, J.K.; Choi, S.W.; Park, C.H.; Kim, S.W.; Kim, S.E.; Reddy, N.S.; Yeom, J.T. Characterization of hot deformation behavior and processing maps of Ti–19Al–22Mo alloy. *Met. Mater. Int.* **2019**, *25*, 1063–1071. [CrossRef]
28. Edwards, T.E.J.; Gioacchino, F.D.; Mohanty, G.; Wehrs, J.; Michler, J.; Clegg, W.J. Longitudinal twinning in a TiAl alloy at high-temperature by, in situ, microcompression. *Acta Mater.* **2018**, *148*, 202–215. [CrossRef]
29. Cheng, L.; Chang, H.; Tang, B.; Kou, H.C.; Li, J.S. Deformation and dynamic recrystallization behavior of a high Nb containing Ti Al alloy. *J. Alloys Compd.* **2013**, *552*, 363–369. [CrossRef]
30. Klein, T.; Rashkova, B.; Holec, D.; Clemens, H.; Mayer, S. Silicon distribution and silicide precipitation during annealing in an advanced multi-phase γ-TiAl based alloy. *Acta Mater.* **2016**, *110*, 236–245. [CrossRef]
31. Su, Y.Q.; Liu, X.W.; Luo, L.S.; Zhao, L.; Guo, J.J.; Fu, H.Z. Hydrogen solubility in molten TiAl alloys. *Int. J. Hydrogen Energy* **2010**, *35*, 8008–8013. [CrossRef]
32. Bode, B.; Wessel, W.; Brueckner-Foit, A.; Mildner, J.; Wollenhaupt, M.; Baument, T. Local deformation at micro-notches and crack initiation in an intermetallic γ-TiAl-alloy. *Fatigue Fract. Eng. Mater. Struct.* **2016**, *39*, 227–237. [CrossRef]

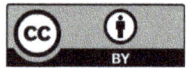

© 2020 by the authors. Licensee MDPI, Basel, Switzerland. This article is an open access article distributed under the terms and conditions of the Creative Commons Attribution (CC BY) license (http://creativecommons.org/licenses/by/4.0/).

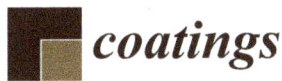

Article

Microstructural and Corrosion Characteristics of Al-Fe Alloys Produced by High-Frequency Induction-Sintering Process

Asiful H. Seikh [1,*], Muneer Baig [2], Jitendra Kumar Singh [3,*], Jabair A. Mohammed [1], Monis Luqman [4], Hany S. Abdo [1,5], Amir Rahman Khan [4] and Nabeel H. Alharthi [4]

1. Centre of Excellence for Research in Engineering Materials, King Saud University, P.O. Box-800, Riyadh 11421, Saudi Arabia; jmohammed@ksu.edu.sa (J.A.M.); habdo@ksu.edu.sa (H.S.A.)
2. Engineering Management Department, College of Engineering, Prince Sultan University, P.O. Box No. 66833 Rafha Street, Riyadh 11586, Saudi Arabia; dr.muneerbaig@gmail.com
3. Innovative Durable Building and Infrastructure Research Center, Department of Architectural Engineering, Hanyang University, 1271 Sa3-dong, Sangrok-gu, Ansan 15588, Korea
4. Mechanical Engineering Department, College of Engineering, King Saud University, P.O. Box-800, Riyadh 11421, Saudi Arabia; monisluqman9@gmail.com (M.L.); aamirk930@gmail.com (A.R.K.); alharthy@ksu.edu.sa (N.H.A.)
5. Mechanical Design and Materials Department, Faculty of Energy Engineering, Aswan University, Aswan 81521, Egypt
* Correspondence: aseikh@ksu.edu.sa (A.H.S.); jk200386@hanyang.ac.kr (J.K.S.); Tel.: +966-1-467-0760 (A.H.S.); +82-31-436-8159 (J.K.S.)

Received: 14 August 2019; Accepted: 18 September 2019; Published: 21 October 2019

Abstract: Al-x wt.% Fe bulk alloys were fabricated from a powder mixture of pure Al and x wt.% of Fe, where x = 2 wt.%, 5 wt.% and 10 wt.%. Initially, as-mixed mixtures were processed using a mechanical-alloying (MA) technique in an attritor for 4 h. The milling was performed in an argon atmosphere at room temperature followed by the sintering of the milled powders in a high-frequency induction furnace to produce bulk samples. Scanning electron microscopy (SEM) was used to study the morphology of the produced alloys, and X-ray diffraction (XRD) to determine the phases formed after the sintering process and their crystallite size. The corrosion behavior of the fabricated samples was studied by immerging them in a 3.5% sodium chloride (NaCl) solution at room temperature using cyclic-polarization (CP) and electrochemical-impedance-spectroscopy (EIS) techniques. The SEM results showed that Fe was uniformly distributed in the Al matrix, and XRD revealed the formation of Al and intermetallic, i.e., Al_6Fe and $Al_{13}Fe_4$, phases in the Al-Fe alloys after sintering. The hardness of the Al-Fe alloys was increased with the addition of Fe due to the formation of intermetallic compounds. Electrochemical results showed that there was a proportional relationship between the percentage of Fe additives and corrosion potential (E_{corr}) where it shifted toward a nobler direction, while corrosion current density (i_{corr}) and corrosion rate decreased with an increasing Fe%. This observation indicates that the addition of Fe into an Al matrix leads to an improvement in the corrosion resistance of the alloys.

Keywords: mechanical alloying; nanocrystalline alloys; corrosion; polarization; EIS

1. Introduction

The mechanical-alloying (MA) technique is used to fabricate bulk metallic alloys from elemental powders that demonstrate better physical and mechanical properties when compared with similar alloys produced using a conventional manufacturing process [1–3]. MA can be defined as a solid-state powder-processing technique. It includes the fabrication of bulk metallic alloys from powder-mixture processes, such as consolidation and sintering, in order to produce a homogeneous structure. It has been reported in the literature that the MA technique leads to the production of stable microstructures in terms of the uniform dispersion of oxides, and produces alloys with fine-grain structures [4]. In the MA process, a high-energy ball mill is usually used due to its simplicity and effectiveness to attain a fine grain size and homogeneous dispersion of the elemental powders in the mixture [5]. However, the process variables in MA are time, types of milling, environment or atmosphere, and ball-to-powder weight ratio. These process variables were reported to have an effect on the powder properties and the structure of the processed powders [6].

Aluminum and its alloys have recently been used in the automotive industry, aerospace and military fields owing to good mechanical properties such as improved strength, hardness, and a high-specificity elastic modulus [7,8]. The addition of 5 wt.% Fe in an Al matrix could lead to improvement in the mechanical properties of the alloys owing to grain refinement and the formation of intermetallic compounds such as Al_6Fe and $Al_{13}Fe_4$ [9]. It was reported that transition metals are not freely miscible in Al, for example, the solubility of Fe in Al can reach the maximum level of 0.03%, which delays the age-hardening process [10,11]. Nonequilibrium processes, such as mechanical-alloying and rapid-solidification techniques, are used to increase the solubility of Fe in an α-Al matrix [12–16]. Alloys with a higher amount of Fe and improved microstructures show a better physical and mechanical properties compared to an alloy of Al with less Fe content [17–20].

The addition of Fe in an Al matrix through the MA process leads to the production of nanocrystalline and amorphous Al-Fe alloys due to the formation of a supersaturated solution [21,22]. Niu et al. produced Al-Fe alloys with MA processing where they reported that by adding 5 wt.% to 12 wt.% Fe can produce excellent tensile strength and stiffness at room and elevated temperatures due to the strengthening of Al by intermetallics as well as to the stabilization of the structure [23]. However, there is limitation to the Fe content that can be dissolved in an Al matrix using the MA process. Nayak et al. reported that, once the amount of Fe content increased by more than 10 wt.% Fe, the alloys suffered from the formation of nonequilibrium intermetallic Al_5Fe_2, which hinders the formation of a supersaturated solution [24]. Once the amount of Fe was increased more than 10 wt.%, the dissolution of Fe decreased and ultimate tensile strength decreased [23]. Thus, it was suggested from the above literature that more than 10 wt.% Fe cannot be used to obtain a supersaturated solution of Al-Fe alloys for application.

Al and their alloys are known to exhibit good corrosion resistance due to the development of an oxide layer on the surface [1,2,8–13,25–30]. However, coarse-grained Al exhibits uniform and pitting corrosion when immersed in acidic or harsh atmospheric conditions [12–14,27,30]. The corrosion resistance of nanocrystalline materials differs from their coarse-grain counterpart due to their smaller crystallite sizes. Additionally, it is known that nanocrystalline materials increase corrosion resistance in passivating environments [31]. A similar study on the nanocrystalline Al-Cr alloy suggested that the Al-Cr alloy showed improvement in its corrosion resistance when compared with the values obtained from pure aluminum [32]. Another study on the addition of nanocrystalline Cu and Ti elements into Al showed improved corrosion resistance [33]. However, the corrosion resistance of nanocrystalline and coarse-grained Al was affected, as it was reported that the formation of pits on the alloy surface resulted in higher corrosion than the values obtained from the coarse-grained material. This could be due to the presence of less grain-boundary volume in coarse-grained materials than nanocrystalline materials [34,35]. Based on several earlier investigations, it was observed that the corrosion behavior of nanocrystalline materials is dependent on several factors, such as alloying element [25], manufacturing process [36,37], microstructure type [38,39] and environmental conditions [40,41].

From the above literature, it was found that there is a lack of information on the effect of Fe addition in an Al matrix using a mechanical-alloying and sintering process in terms of morphological and corrosion characteristics. In the present study, we fabricated Al and Al-Fe alloys with the incorporation of 2 wt.%, 5 wt.%, and 10 wt.% Fe using an MA technique followed by the sintering process. The morphological and corrosion characteristics of fabricated alloys were carried out by immerging them in a 3.5% NaCl solution for 1 h via cyclic-polarization (CP) and electrochemical-impedance-spectroscopy (EIS) techniques.

2. Materials and Methods

2.1. Fabrication of Pure Al and Al-Fe Alloys

Raw powders of Al (99.95% purity) and Fe (99.95% purity) were used to fabricate the alloys. The average particle size of Al was 5 μm, while the Fe (initial size = 45 μm) was premilled to achieve an average particle size of 13 μm. Before milling, pure Al and a proportionate mixture of premilled Fe (2 wt.%, 5 wt.%, and 10 wt.%) were degassed at 453 K for 24 h under vacuum. The mechanical alloying was carried out in an attritor (Figure 1) with a 5 mm stainless steel ball. The ball-to-powder weight ratio was 30:1 along with 1% of stearic acid powder (process-control agent). The balls and degassed-powder mixtures with the stearic acid were charged into the steel canister (container) of the attritor at 100 rpm, and the speed of the attritor was gradually increased to 250 rpm. Mechanical alloying (Al-2 wt.%, Al-5 wt.%, and Al-10 wt.% Fe) was performed in an inert atmosphere for 4 h. In order to maintain a constant temperature inside the attritor canister (container), we gave a 15 min pause for every 30 min of milling that was followed by a continuous supply of cold water in the outer chamber of the canister.

Finally, bulk samples were obtained by the consolidation and sintering of the milled powders. The milled powders were transferred into a graphite die in a vacuum glove box and pressed using a hydraulic jack to produce a green body. After pressing for 15 min, the graphite die was transferred to a high-frequency induction sintering (I IFIS, ELTek, Seoul, Korea) machine. The machine chamber was set to vacuum, the powder was further pressed in the HFIS machine to 100 MPa, and the sintering temperature was set to 823 K. The pressing was continued for 6 min at 823 K. After 6 min of loading, the graphite die was allowed to cool in the HFIS chamber. Later, the sample was removed from the die to obtain the bulk alloys.

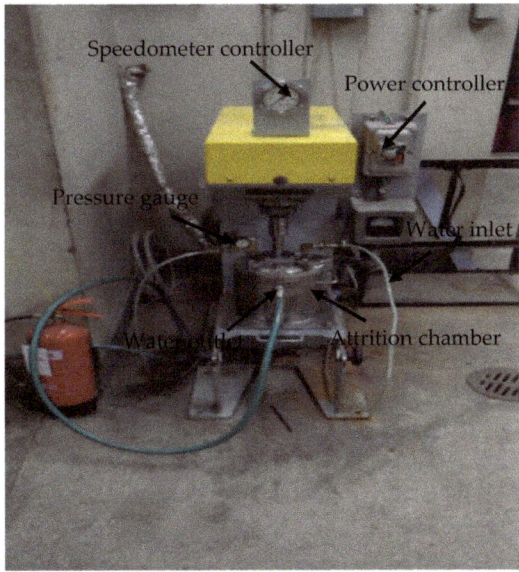

Figure 1. Attritor.

2.2. Characterization Using X-ray Diffraction (XRD)

XRD (Bruker, Hamburg, Germany) analysis of the fabricated alloys and corrosion products was performed using Cu-Kα (λ = 0.154 nm) radiation. For the XRD peak profile, the data were captured within 2θ = 20°–90°. Peak-profile data were used to determine the crystallite size and microstrain of the sintered bulk samples using the Williamson–Hall method [42,43].

2.3. Microstructure Characterization of Sintered Alloys

Microstructural characterization of the polished-sintered-alloy surface (pure Al, Al-2 wt.%, Al-5 wt.%, and Al-10 wt.% Fe) and the corroded samples was carried out using a field emission scanning electron microscope (FESEM, JOEL, Tokyo, Japan). Elemental analysis of the alloys was obtained using an energy-dispersive spectrometry (EDS) analyzer attached to the FESEM device. Grain-size analysis of the alloys was carried out with ImageJ software (version 1.52n).

2.4. Hardness Measurement

To evaluate the Vickers hardness of the fabricated materials, a WOLPERT UH930 Universal Hardness Testing Machine (Lieca VMHT Auto, Tokyo, Japan) was employed. The load was 10 kgf and dwell time was 10 s. Hardness measurement was repeated for 5 readings, and the average was taken to represent the hardness value.

2.5. Electrochemical Cell

Electrochemical experiments were performed using three electrode systems consisting of a platinum foil as the counter electrode (CE), Ag/AgCl as the reference electrode (RE), and the fabricated sintered alloys were selected as the working electrode (WE). A solution of 3.5% NaCl (analytical-grade reagents) was prepared in distilled water for the electrochemical experiments. WE preparation and mounting was performed using a standard procedure and can be found elsewhere [44]. WE was fabricated by making a 0.5 mm hole in depth, and the same diameter was drilled into one surface. A copper wire of the same diameter was placed and soldered. This assembly was mounted in an epoxy resin and kept for 24 h to cure at room temperature. After drying, the sample was polished with 1200 μm emery paper, then alumina (0.5 μm particle size) slurry to obtain a smooth surface using an automatic polishing machine (Buehler MetaServ 250, Shanghai, China).

2.6. Electrochemical Experiments

Electrochemical experiments of pure Al, Al-2 wt.%, Al-5 wt.%, and Al-10 wt.% Fe alloys were performed with an Autolab system (PGSTAT20, Metrohm, Barendrecht, The Netherlands) by immerging them in 3.5% NaCl solution. For every new experiment, a new polished surface was prepared for each electrode, and fresh 3.5% NaCl solution was used. The CP experiment was performed by changing the potential from −1200 to +0.00 mV at a scan rate of 1 mV/s, alongside the RE from open-circuit potential (OCP). EIS was measured within a frequency variation from 0.0001 to 100 kHz with 10 steps per decade by applying 5 mV sinusoidal perturbation at the OCP.

3. Results and Discussion

The SEM micrographs with the corresponding EDS analysis (arrow mark in respective figures) of pure Al and Al-10 wt.% Fe alloys after the sintering process are shown in Figure 2a,b, respectively. No porosity is shown in the SEM micrographs of pure Al (Figure 2a) or the Al-10 wt.% Fe alloys (Figure 2b), which indicates the perfect fabrication process with HFIS, as confirmed by the high relative-density values (>98%) of the sintered samples. Pure Al showed 100% Al in the EDS result (Figure 2a) which confirm that there no oxidation occurred during the HFIS process. Due to mixing 10 wt.% Fe in the alloy, dispersion of fine Fe particles in Al matrix was shown with uniform intermetallic distribution [23], as shown in Figure 2b. From this figure, it can be observed that the Fe was completely mixed and uniformly distributed in the Al matrix; thus, there was no segregation found [45]. On the basis of the Al-10 wt.% Fe alloy microstructure, it is possible to say that it formed a homogeneous and uniform mixture without porosity, which may improve the microstructural stability of fabricated alloys.

On the basis of EDS analysis (respective particle analysis shown by arrow marks in Figure 2b), the white contrast contained 64 wt.% Al and 34 wt.% Fe, and their probable stoichiometric formula would be very close to $Al_{13}Fe_4$. The gray contrast contained 73.27 wt.% Al and 26.73 wt.% Fe, and its probable stoichiometric formula would be close to Al_6Fe. On the other hand, the black contrast was almost Al, where it contained 99.30% Al, which was the α-Al reported by Sasaki et al. [9]. This result suggests that Fe was completely mixed into the Al matrix after the attrition and sintering process. Overall EDS analysis showed 90 wt.% Al and 10 wt.% Fe, which is a parent material composition (90 wt.% Al and 10 wt.% Fe). Phase verification by XRD analysis is described in the subsequent paragraph to corroborate the EDS results. The grain size of Al, $Al_{13}Fe_4$, and Al_6Fe was found to be around 430 ± 27, 490 ± 15, and 604 ± 32 nm, respectively, in the Al-10 wt.% Fe alloys.

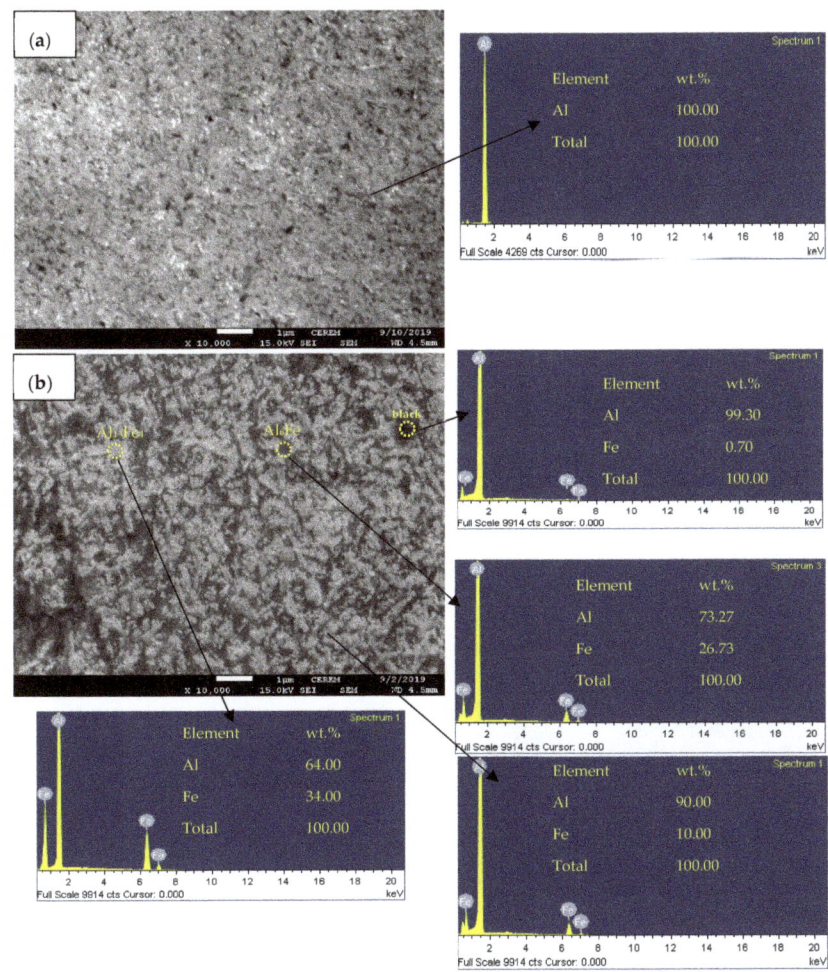

Figure 2. Scanning-electron-microscopy (SEM) micrograph and corresponding energy-dispersive-spectrometry (EDS) pattern of (**a**) pure Al and (**b**) Al-10 wt.% Fe alloys after sintering process.

The X-ray diffraction patterns for the pure Al and Al-10 wt.% Fe alloys are shown in Figure 3. For the pure Al sample, the observed diffraction peaks corresponded to (111), (200), (220), and (222) planes of α-Al (JCPS = 85-1327). Peak broadening (after milling and sintering) along with a peak-intensity (height) decrease was observed in the Al-10 wt.% Fe alloys. This might be due to enhanced crystal-size refinement, it being amorphous, and the formation of new intermetallic compounds during MA process with addition of Fe [24]. In Al-10 wt.% Fe alloy-diffraction peaks,

Al$_6$Fe (JCPS = 47-1433) and Al$_{13}$Fe$_4$ (JCPS = 29-0042), along with the main α-Al peaks, were identified as intermetallic compounds. The formation of intermetallic compounds corroborates the EDS analysis results. These new intermetallic compounds were obtained because, during the milling process, the added Fe was completely mixed with Al and formed a uniform mixture of Al-Fe alloys. During the sintering process, Fe from the mixture was expelled as part of the new intermetallic compounds due to high temperature and pressure. The formation of these new Al$_6$Fe and Al$_{13}$Fe$_4$ intermetallic compounds occurred during the sintering process at the relatively high temperature of 823 K. Moreover, the presence of Al$_6$Fe and Al$_{13}$Fe$_4$ intermetallic compounds in the fabricated alloys enhanced the mechanical properties and improved the microstructural stability of the sintered alloys.

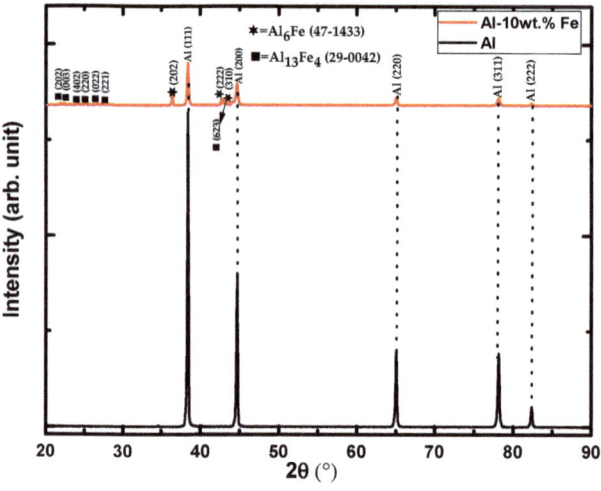

Figure 3. X-ray diffraction (XRD) pattern for pure Al and Al-10 wt.% Fe after sintering.

Based on the X-ray diffraction pattern shown in Figure 3, crystallite size and microstrain were calculated from peak width using the linear Williamson–Hall method [42]. Average crystallite size, microstrain, and error were determined for all Al peaks [43]. Table 1 shows crystallite sizes for all alloys used in this investigation. The crystallite sizes of the Al phase in pure Al, Al-2 wt.% Fe, Al-5 wt.% Fe, and Al-10 wt.% Fe were found to be 53.67 ± 1.78, 39.16 ± 4.23, 39.13 ± 2.70, and 37.33 ± 3.56 nm, respectively (Table 1). It was observed that the crystallite size of the Al phase was decreased and the microstrain gradually increased as Fe content was increased in the Al-Fe alloys. In the case of the addition of Fe of more than 10 wt.% to the Al matrix, the microstrain was increased and resulted in the formation of a brittle surface due to the extreme refinement of the crystallite [24]. Thus, this study did not allow Fe content to increase by more than 10 wt.% Fe. This observation may also be explained on the basis of intermetallic-compound formation that hinders grain growth during the sintering process, thereby leading to a uniform and stable microstructure in the fabricated alloys.

Table 1. Alloy crystallite size and microstrain.

Materials	Crystallite Size (Error), nm	Microstrain (Error), %
Pure Al	53.67 ± 1.78	0.17 ± 0.05
Al-2 wt.% Fe	39.16 ± 4.23	0.22 ± 0.03
Al-5 wt.% Fe	39.13 ± 2.70	0.23 ± 0.04
Al-10 wt.% Fe	37.33 ± 3.56	0.24 ± 0.04

The volume fraction (V_f) of Al and the intermetallic compounds present in Al and Al-10 wt.% Fe alloys was calculated based on the integrated-surface-area method [46–49]:

$$V_{f(Al)} = \frac{A_{Al}}{A_{Al} + A_{Al_{13}Fe_4} + A_{Al_6Fe}} \quad (1)$$

$$V_{f(Al_{13}Fe_4)} = \frac{A_{Al_{13}Fe_4}}{A_{Al} + A_{Al_{13}Fe_4} + A_{Al_6Fe}} \quad (2)$$

$$V_{f(Al_6Fe)} = \frac{A_{Al_6Fe}}{A_{Al} + A_{Al_{13}Fe_4} + A_{Al_6Fe}} \quad (3)$$

where $V_{f(Al)}$, $V_{f(Al_{13}Fe_4)}$, and $V_{f(Al_6Fe)}$ were volume fractions, and A_{Al}, $A_{Al_{13}Fe_4}$, and A_{Al_6Fe} were the total integrated surface area of Al, $Al_{13}Fe_4$, and A_6Fe, respectively. Based on the above calculation, $V_{f(Al)}$ in pure Al was found to be 100% due to the presence of only one phase, while in Al-10 wt.% Fe alloys, $V_{f(Al)}$, $V_{f(Al_{13}Fe_4)}$, and $V_{f(Al_6Fe)}$ showed 81.78%, 2.32%, and 15.90%, respectively.

Figure 4 shows the compressive stress–strain response of all fabricated alloys. The experiment was performed at a strain rate of 0.0001/sec at room temperature. From the results, it was evident that the strength of the alloys was increased with an increase in the amount of alloying element (Fe). However, elongation to failure was decreased. This result was expected because, as the strength of an alloy increases, then its elongation to failure decreases.

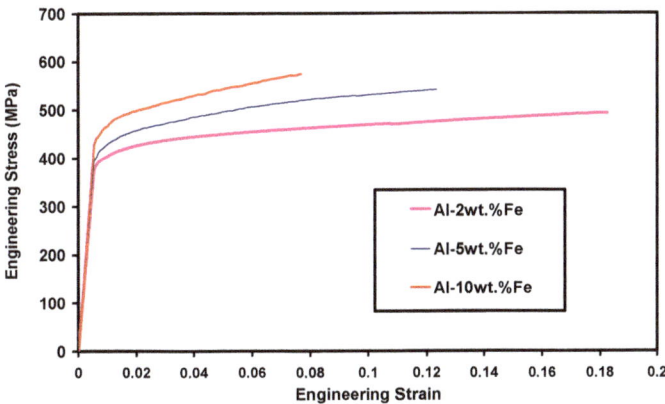

Figure 4. Compressive stress–strain response of Al-Fe fabricated alloys.

Alloy hardness with error is shown in Figure 5. As the amount of Fe increased, the hardness of the Al-Fe alloys also significantly increased owing to the formation of nanocrystalline Al-Fe alloys with crystallite/grain refinement [50]. The hardness of Al, Al-2 wt.% Fe, Al-5 wt.% Fe, and Al-10 wt.% Fe was found to be 44.87, 97.55, 110.75, and 135.03 HV, respectively. Once the 10 wt.% Fe was added in Al, hardness was increased by more than 200%. This phenomenon occurred due to the influence of grain-size refinement, where crystallite size is decreased after the addition of Fe in Al [51]. It is well known that the hardness of intermetallic compounds, especially Al_6Fe, is greater than that of pure metals or alloys [52,53]. Alloy hardness can be correlated with intermetallic volume fraction calculated with XRD, where Al-10 wt.% Fe alloys contain 2.32% $Al_{13}Fe_4$ and 15.90% Al_6Fe, which play an important role in hardness enhancement.

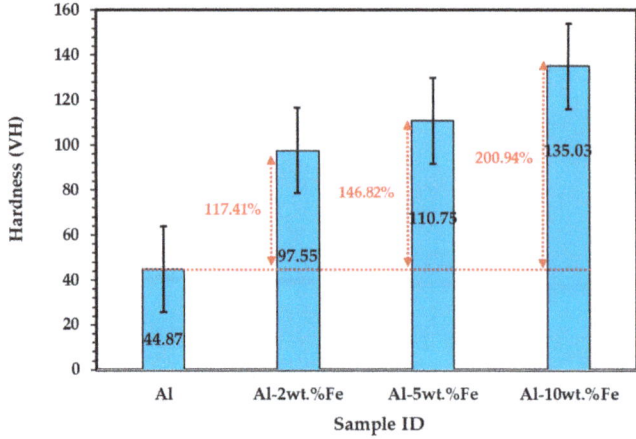

Figure 5. Hardness of Al and Al-Fe fabricated alloys.

To confirm the uniform dispersion of Fe particles in the Al matrix, EDS elemental mapping was performed using FESEM on the surface of the Al-10 wt.% Fe sintered sample, as shown in Figure 6. EDS mapping of the Al-10 wt.% Fe alloys (Figure 6a) clearly indicated homogeneous dispersion in gray and black contrast due to the presence of Al and Fe/intermetallic compounds [54]. The black contrast represents Al distribution, since it was represented in the SEM image (Figure 2b), while the gray contrast surrounded the Al matrix by the formation of Fe/intermetallic compounds [9]. The bright-yellow contrast in Figure 6b represents Al, and the dark contrast indicates Fe/intermetallic presence. Similarly, in Figure 6c, it can be seen that the blue contrast represents the presence of Fe particles, while the black and white particles show intermetallic presence. From EDS mapping, it was clear that Fe particles were homogeneously distributed in the Al matrix of Al-10 wt.% Fe alloys.

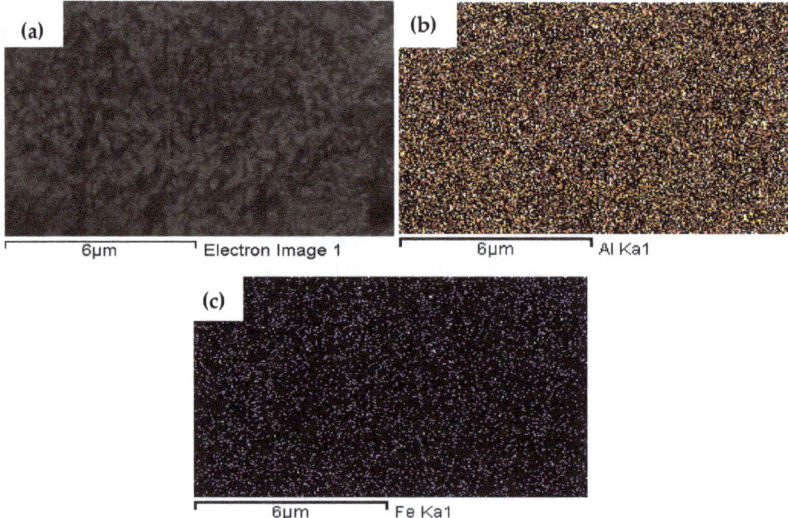

Figure 6. (a) EDS mapping of Al-10 wt.% Fe sintered sample, (b) elemental mapping showing location and presence of Al, and (c) elemental mapping showing location and presence of Fe.

3.1. Electrochemical Measurements

CP was used to examine the corrosion resistance of Al and Al-Fe sintered alloys by immerging them in 3.5% NaCl solution for one hour. The CP results of the fabricated alloys are shown in Figure 7. Electrochemical parameters such as corrosion current density (i_{corr}), corrosion potential (E_{corr}), pitting potential (E_{pit}), pitting current (i_{pit}), and polarization resistance (R_p) were extracted after fitting the polarization curves in Tafel's regions; results are shown in Table 2. All samples showed positive (clockwise) loop formation during the back scanning, which revealed alloy deterioration.

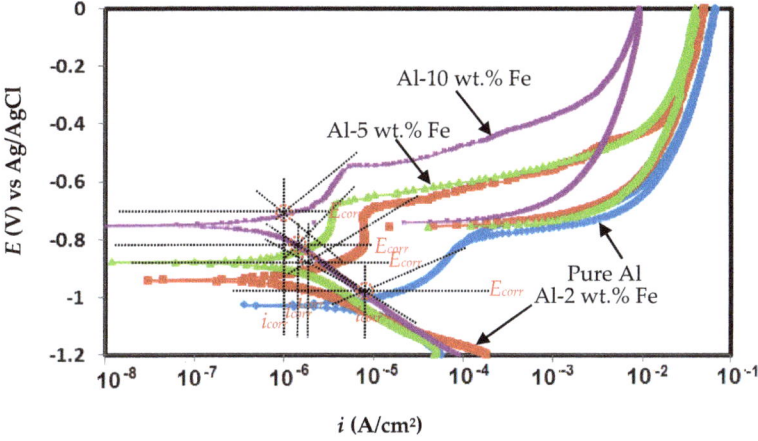

Figure 7. Cyclic-polarization (CP) curves for pure Al and Al-Fe alloys after one hour immersion in 3.5% NaCl solution.

Table 2. Electrochemical parameters obtained after fitting CP graphs in Tafel regions for pure Al and Al-Fe alloys after one hour immersion in 3.5% NaCl solution.

Materials	Electrochemical Parameters					
	E_{corr} (mV) vs Ag/AgCl	i_{corr} ($\mu A \cdot cm^{-2}$)	E_{pit} (mV) vs Ag/AgCl	i_{pit} ($\mu A \cdot cm^{-2}$)	R_p (k$\Omega \cdot cm^2$)	Corrosion Rate (μm/year)
Pure Al	−1047	14.48	−824	89.3	4.873	157.83
Al-2 wt.% Fe	−940	1.35	−714	8.43	21.58	14.77
Al-5 wt.% Fe	−884	1.27	−698	4.64	38.23	14.38
Al-10 wt.% Fe	−752	1.05	−569	4.48	53.05	11.63

The CP curve showed the active–passive behavior of the pure Al as well as the binary Al-Fe alloys. It was observed that the addition of Fe resulted in an increase in cathodic current density owing to the presence of greater intermetallic compounds that worked as cathode sites where hydrogen-evolution reaction occurred [55,56]. Moreover, cathodic current density was increased once Fe content was increased in the Al-Fe alloys. Pure Al showed a sudden increment in current density after E_{corr}, which showed pitting, whereas, once the Fe was added in the Al-Fe alloys, it formed a passive film after E_{corr}. The formation of a passive film in the Al-Fe alloys at lower current density revealed protection against corrosion in the NaCl solution. Passivation was observed once Fe was incorporated in the Al-Fe alloys during anodic scanning at a different current density due to the formation of intermetallic compounds in alloys such as $Al_{13}Fe_4$ and Al (Fe), which is correlated with the results of Flores-Chan et al., where they found that Al-Fe (20 wt.%) alloys facilitate forming a passive film [57]. It was observed by other researchers that the corrosion protection of Al–Fe alloys is due to the formation of stable passive films (ferrous and aluminum hydroxide/aluminum ions) exposed to NaCl solution owing to the preferential dissolution of $FeAl_3$ [54,58].

The corrosion rate of Al and Al-Fe alloys was calculated using the following equation [59]:

$$\text{Corrosion rate (μm/year)} = \frac{3.27 \times i_{corr} \times E.W.}{d} \quad (4)$$

The corrosion rate in Equation (4) is expressed in μm/year, while i_{corr} is in units of μA·cm^{-2}. The value of i_{corr} was obtained by dividing the total surface area of the working electrode in the corrosion current. E.W. represents the equivalent weight (g/mole), and d is the density (g/cm^3) of the alloys.

The potential, such as E_{corr} and E_{pit} values, shifted toward a more positive direction once Fe was added in the Al-Fe alloys, which shows it to be nobler in nature (Table 2). It was also reported that anodic currents, i_{corr} and i_{pit} values decreased and R_p values increased with the increase of the amount of Fe in an Al alloy. The positive influence of Fe addition in regards to the corrosion resistance of Al-Fe alloys is due to the presence of intermetallic compounds. The increase in R_p value and decrease in i_{corr} of the fabricated alloys could be accredited to three facts: first, the presence of secondary intermetallic phases, i.e., Al$_6$Fe and Al$_{13}$Fe$_4$, in the alloy, as observed in the XRD of the sintered sample. Second, the formation of a homogeneous mixture due to alloying is known to improve the microstructural stability of an alloy and improve its corrosion resistance. Third, the increase in R_p value might also be due to the formation of passive layers of Al$_2$O$_3$ and Fe$_2$O$_3$ on the alloy surface of the exposed samples [60]. Additionally, Al dissociation decreased structural stability; thus, it impeded complex aluminum chloride formation, which initiates pitting corrosion [61].

The corrosion characteristics of pure Al and Al-Fe alloys were studied using the EIS technique to determine their kinetics and mechanism. The corrosion behavior of pure Al and Al-Fe alloy samples was examined in a 3.5% NaCl solution at room temperature after one hour of exposure. The Nyquist plots obtained at OCP are shown in Figure 8.

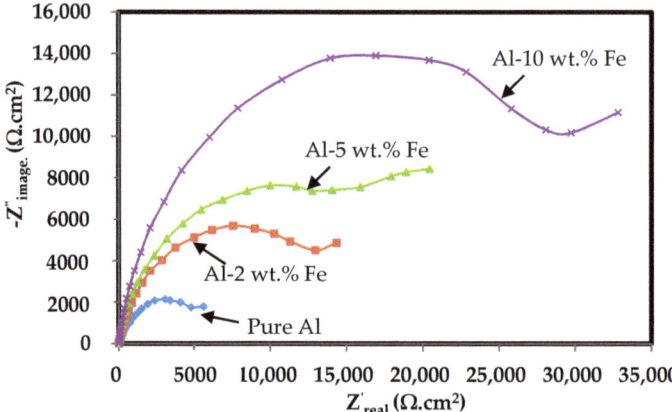

Figure 8. Nyquist plot for pure Al and Al-Fe alloys after one hour of immersion in 3.5% NaCl solution.

Two types of semicircle loops are shown in the Nyquist plot (Figure 8), a half semicircle loop in a low-frequency range and a capacitive loop at a high-frequency range, which could be due to the charge–transfer reaction (corrosion-product activity as a passive layer) between electrolyte and alloy interface via the electrochemical twin layer. However, the low-frequency loop could be related to the corrosion characteristics of alloys.

The suitable equivalent circuit model (ECM) is shown in Figure 9 to fit EIS plots and extract the kinetics parameters. This ECM contained two circuits, where the first circuit contained charge transfer resistance (R_{ct}) at the electrode/solution interface and the double-layer capacitance (C_{dl}), which were parallel with each other. Another circuit contained the layer resistance that was inter-related with the resistance of the corrosion film (R_f) and the capacitance of the film (C_f), which were parallel with each other. R_{ct} with R_f and C_{dl} with C_f were connected in series with each other. The first circuit represented the corrosion characteristics of the alloys, whereas the second was for film formation at the alloy/solution interface. From the ECM (Figure 8), calculation of electrochemical impedance parameters such as solution resistance (R_s), R_{ct}, C_{dl}, R_f, and C_f was obtained [62]. Table 3 shows the value of these calculated parameters. In order to give a more accurate fitting, constant phase elements (CPE) were replaced for the capacitive elements of the corrosion film (CPE_f or C_f), pseudocapacitance and double-layer capacitance (CPE_{dl} or C_{dl}). For various corrosion parameters, it is well known that R_{ct} is the factor that expresses the corrosion behavior of alloys, and its value is inversely proportional to i_{corr}.

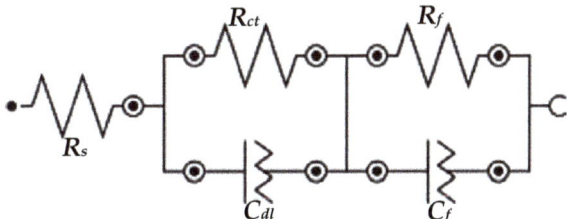

Figure 9. Equivalent circuit model (ECM) for EIS.

Table 3. Electrochemical-impedance-spectroscopy (EIS) parameters for pure Al and Al-Fe alloys after one hour of immersion in 3.5% NaCl solution.

Materials	R_S (Ω·cm²)	Q1		R_{ct} (kΩ·cm²)	Q2		R_f (kΩ·cm²)
		C_{dl} (μF·cm⁻²)	n		C_f (μF·cm⁻²)	n	
Pure Al	3.84	248.3	0.977	1.11	617	0.58	2.81
Al-2% Fe	11.5	15.4	0.778	7.12	37.6	0.884	9.6
Al-5% Fe	13.8	12.8	0.887	11.1	23.4	0.92	13.6
Al-10% Fe	22.1	10.1	0.843	21.5	13.6	0.862	35.0

It was noted from the Nyquist plot that increasing the Fe amount in the alloy led to a proportional increase in the diameter of the arc/loop at both axes (Z'_{real} and $-Z''_{image}$), which indicated that, by increasing the amount of Fe, corrosion resistance of an Al-Fe alloy was increased. From Table 3, it can be concluded that, by increasing the amount of Fe in the alloy, there is a proportional increase in the values of both R_{ct} and R_f and a decrease in C_{dl} and C_f. Higher values of R_{ct} mean a substantial rise in the corrosion-resistance values of the alloy, and they are attributed to the development of an oxide layer on the surface of the fabricated Al-Fe alloys.

The expression that defines the impedance of the CPE is: $Z_{CPE} = 1/Y (j\omega)$, where $j^2 = -1$ represents an imaginary number and n is referred to as the CPE exponent, which varies, $-1 < n < 1$; angular frequency (in rad s⁻¹) is represented by ω; and Y is the CPE constant. It was reported earlier that CPEs can be assumed to be resistance, capacitance, or inductance, depending on the value of n [63]. In the current study, CPE_{dl} specifies the twin-layer capacitors as values of n varying between 0.78 and 0.98. When the n was lower than 0.78, then it indicated that the passive layer developed on the surface was porous and nonuniform [64]. Additionally, when n was lower than 0.51–0.61, then CPE_f represents Warburg impedance (W). The corrosion resistance of Al alloys in 3.5% NaCl is attributed to the formation of oxide film and/or corrosion products on the surface [65]. It was noted that R_{ct} was lower than the value of R_f, which signified that the inner layer worked as barrier that caused resistance for corrosion protection [66]. In this investigation, EIS measurements were consistent with the trend obtained from the CP data. Both of these techniques confirm that the Al-10 wt.% Fe alloy had the highest corrosion resistance from all alloys in the 3.5% NaCl solution due to the formation of compact, adherent, and protective passive films on its surface.

The Bode-phase diagram was obtained during the EIS experiments of the pure Al and Al-Fe alloys after one hour of immersion in 3.5% NaCl solution, and the results are shown in Figure 10. It is clearly observed from this figure that total impedance values were gradually increased once the amount of Fe was increased from 2 wt.% to 10 wt.% at 0.1 Hz. As the Fe amount was increased up to 10 wt.%, corrosion resistance, i.e., total obtained impedance, was the highest due to the presence of the highest intermetallic amount in the Al-10 wt.% Fe alloys, which facilitated the formation of a passive film. It was concluded that the Al-10 wt.% Fe alloy had the highest impedance value; therefore, it gave the best resistance against corrosion. This trend implies that there was a proportional relation between increasing the percentage of iron content in the Al matrix and the corrosion resistance of the Al-Fe alloys.

Capacitive behavior due to the presence of two time constants, typically as in passive materials, can be clearly noticed from the Bode plot (Figure 10). The phase angle was shifted from −60° for pure Al to −80° for Al-10 wt.% Fe at a middle studied frequency, which revealed the capacitive properties of the film. Shifting in phase-angle maxima in a broad range of middle frequency at −80° revealed that, after exposure to the NaCl solution, the surface became homogeneous and resistive due to the formation of a passive film. This result indicates that there formed a thin, stable layer at the alloy/solution interface that covered the surface of the Al-Fe alloys. Pure Al showed phase-angle maxima at −60°, suggesting that the surface became nonhomogeneous and defective; thus, corrosion resistance was the lowest among all samples.

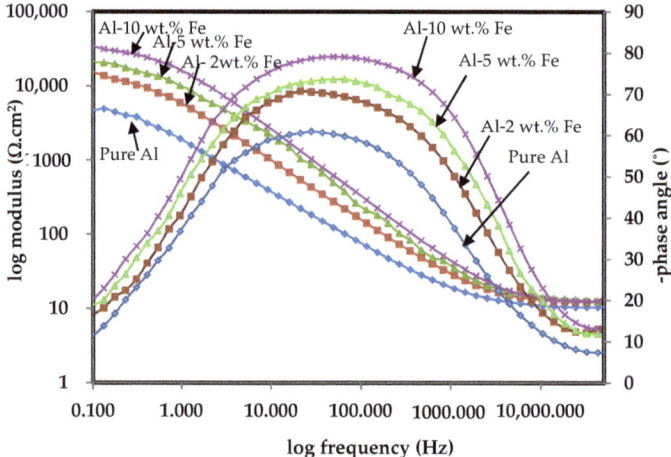

Figure 10. Bode plot for pure Al and Al-Fe alloys after one hour immersion in 3.5% NaCl at room temperature.

3.2. Characterization of Corroded Alloys

SEM micrographs of the corroded pure Al sample surface after one hour of immersion in 3.5% NaCl solution are shown in Figure 11a. This figure indicates that the Al sample surface was mostly corroded with pit formation as well as flakes and crackers due to the localized attack of chloride ion on the Al matrix [67]. Pit formation on the surface was correlated with the CP results where anodic current density increased dramatically after E_{corr}. EDS analysis (arrow mark from Figure 11a) showed 76.74% Al, 10.21% O, 5.38% Na, and 7.67% Cl on the corroded surface. The reduction in the amount of Al from 100% to 76.74% was due to the deterioration of the pure Al sample. The most possibly corrosive product was the development of an aluminum oxide/hydroxide layer with NaCl deposition on the surface. Aluminum oxide/hydroxide layer acts like a protection film that protects the surface from corrosion.

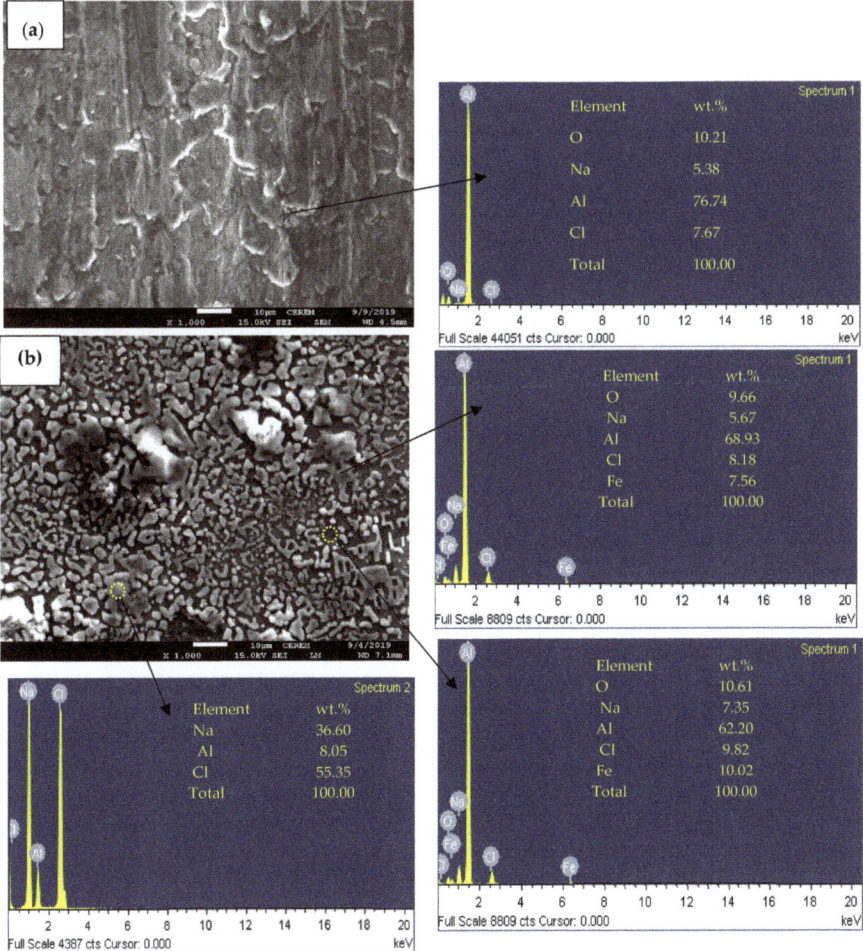

Figure 11. Field emission scanning electron microscope (FESEM) micrographs and EDS profile analysis obtained for (**a**) pure Al and (**b**) Al-10 wt.% Fe alloys after one hour immersion in 3.5% NaCl at room temperature.

SEM images and EDS analysis of the Al-10 wt.% Fe alloys after corrosion are shown in Figure 11b. Corrosion products are regularly deposited over the alloy surface. EDS analysis (arrow mark from Figure 11b) showed 68.93% Al, 7.56% Fe, 9.66% O, 5.67% Na, and 8.18% Cl in wt.% on the surface, which represent corrosion products, while analysis before the corrosion experiment showed it was 90% Al and 10% Fe. The reduction in the amount of Al and Fe after exposure in the NaCl solution suggested that Al and Fe deteriorated where their amount was reduced to around 23% and 24%, respectively, due to the formation of corrosion products on the surface. The presence of a high amount of oxygen in corrosion products proved that a thick corrosion layer was formed that covered the entire alloy surface. The white particles in corrosion products (Figure 11b) were mostly Na and Cl, which revealed the presence of NaCl (from the solution) deposited onto the surface of the Al-10 wt.% Fe alloys.

In the current study, due to the presence of many active centers and the large surface area in the pure Al sample, the reported corrosion-resistance value was lower than that of the Al-Fe alloys. Corrosion-resistance improvement in the Al-Fe alloys was attributed to the combined effect of alloying (Fe addition) and the usage of high-energy ball milling. The ball-milling process extended the mixing of Fe in Al and produced a homogeneous mixture of Al-Fe alloys that hindered pitting corrosion and its influencing abilities for passivation [68]. Corrosion resistance can be improved by mixing Fe in Al, which increases passivation kinetics, stabilizes the passive film, and decreases the difference between the intermetallic bonds and the electrochemical characteristics of the matrix [69].

Consequently, from the characterization information of the fabricated alloys, it was confirmed that the addition of Fe passivated the Al to a higher level by minimizing both pitting and uniform corrosion. By increasing Fe by up to 10 wt.% as an alloying element to Al, the corrosion behavior of the alloy was proportionally enhanced.

The XRD results of corrosion products formed on the pure Al and Al-10 wt.% Fe alloys, along with the respective diffraction patterns and JCPDS number, are shown in Figure 12, which clearly indicates the existence of multiple phases. Pure Al showed Al, α-Al(OH)$_3$ (Bayerite, JCPDS: 83-2256) and NaCl (JCPDS: 88-2300). The Al-10 wt.% Fe alloys contained intermetallic compounds (Al$_{13}$Fe$_4$ and Al$_6$Fe) along with Al, α-Al(OH)$_3$, γ-Fe$_2$O$_3$ (maghemite, JCPDS: 39-1346), and NaCl. The formation of NaCl in the corrosion products of pure Al and Al-10 wt.% Fe came from the studied solution that was deposited onto the surface. From the XRD results of the corrosion products formed on the Al-10 wt.% Fe alloys, it can be found that the number of Al$_6$Fe peaks are identical as those present after the attrition and sintering process (Figure 3), whereas some Al$_{13}$Fe$_4$ peaks disappeared in the corrosion products, which might be attributed to the transformation of Al$_{13}$Fe$_4$ into γ-Fe$_2$O$_3$ and α-Al(OH)$_3$. Intermetallic Al$_6$Fe is very stable and does not allow itself to be dissolved, whereas Al$_{13}$Fe$_4$ facilitates preferential dissolution [67] and is transformed into a stable form of oxide/hydroxide (γ-Fe$_2$O$_3$ and α-Al(OH)$_3$) in NaCl solution. γ-Fe$_2$O$_3$ and α-Al(OH)$_3$ are thermodynamically stable phases of iron oxides and aluminum hydroxide, respectively. It was also reported by other researchers that Al-Fe alloys provide protection against corrosion due to the formation of iron and aluminum hydroxide/oxide as a passive film exposed to NaCl solution [54,58]. Al-10 wt.% Fe alloys provide protection to corrosion due to the presence of γ-Fe$_2$O$_3$ as well as α-Al(OH)$_3$ as corrosion products, which are protective, adherent, and stable in nature. A pure Al corrosion product, on the other hand, showed an absence of γ-Fe$_2$O$_3$. Thus, the corrosion resistance of Al-10 wt.% Fe was greater than that of pure Al in NaCl solution. XRD data of the corrosion products correlate with SEM and EDS results, which leads us to conclude that Al-10 wt.% Fe alloys show the presence of an oxide/hydroxide layer/film on the surface leading to an enhancement of corrosion resistance.

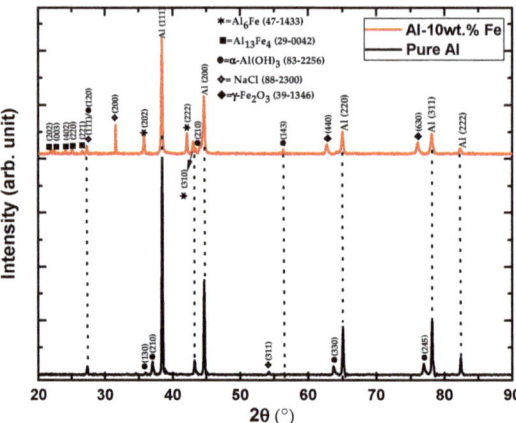

Figure 12. XRD pattern of pure Al and Al-10 wt.% Fe alloys after 1 h of exposure in 3.5% NaCl solution.

4. Conclusions

Using a powder-metallurgy scheme, Al with zero (pure), 2 wt.%, 5 wt.%, and 10 wt.% Fe in Al were successfully fabricated in two-step processes, the MA technique for mixing followed by HFIS for consolidation. The following conclusions can be drawn from the present study:

- Uniform distribution of Fe in an Al matrix was revealed by FESEM and EDS mapping, achieved by the combined process of MA and HFIS.
- XRD results confirmed that as the Fe amount was increased in the Al-Fe alloys, intermetallic-compound, i.e., Al_6Fe and $Al_{13}Fe_4$, formation was increased.
- The presence of intermetallic compounds enhanced the hardness of the Al-Fe alloys due to the influence of grain-size refinement, where the crystallite size was decreased after the addition of Fe in Al.
- Addition of Fe in the Al matrix facilitated the formation of a passive film in the NaCl solution as well as the dramatic decrease of the corrosion rate compared to pure Al.
- EIS studies confirmed that the improved R_{ct} and R_f in Al-Fe alloys compared to pure Al was due to the formation of a protective film on the alloy surface.
- SEM micrographs of the corrosion products formed on the Al-10 wt.% Fe alloys exhibited regular deposition, while pure Al showed pits, craters, and flakes due to the localized attack of chloride ions on the surface.
- XRD results of the corrosion products confirmed the formation of $\gamma\text{-}Fe_2O_3$ and $\alpha\text{-}Al(OH)_3$ on the Al-10 wt.% Fe alloys, which are protective, adherent, and stable in nature, whereas pure Al corrosion products showed an absence of $\gamma\text{-}Fe_2O_3$.

Author Contributions: Conceptualization, A.H.S.; data curation, J.K.S., J.A.M. and H.S.A.; formal analysis, J.K.S., M.B., J.A.M. and H.S.A.; funding acquisition, A.H.S. and N.H.A.; investigation, A.H.S. and M.B.; methodology, J.A.M., M.L., A.R.K. and H.S.A.; resources, N.H.A.; supervision, A.H.S. and N.H.A.; writing—original draft, A.H.S., J.K.S., J.A.M., M.L., A.R.K., M.B., H.S.A. and N.H.A.; writing—review and editing, A.H.S., J.K.S., M.L., A.R.K., M.B., J.A.M., H.S.A. and N.H.A.

Funding: This research received no external funding.

Acknowledgments: The authors would like to extend their sincere appreciation to the Deanship of Scientific Research at King Saud University for its funding of this research through Research Group Project No. RG-1439-029.

Conflicts of Interest: The authors declare no conflict of interest.

References

1. Froes, F.H.; Pickens, J.R. Powder metallurgy of light metal alloys for demanding applications. *JOM J. Miner. Met. Mater. Soc.* **1984**, *36*, 14–28. [CrossRef]
2. Pickens, J.R. Aluminium powder metallurgy technology for high-strength applications. *J. Mater. Sci.* **1981**, *16*, 1437–1457. [CrossRef]
3. Suryanarayana, C. Mechanical alloying and milling. *Prog. Mater. Sci.* **2001**, *46*, 1–184. [CrossRef]
4. Lyle, J.P.; Cebulak, W.S. Powder metallurgy approach for control of microstructure and properties in high strength aluminum alloys. *Metall. Trans. A* **1975**, *6*, 685. [CrossRef]
5. Prabhu, B.; Suryanarayana, C.; An, L.; Vaidyanathan, R. Synthesis and characterization of high volume fraction Al-Al_2O_3 nanocomposite powders by high-energy milling. *Mater. Sci. Eng. A* **2006**, *425*, 192–200. [CrossRef]
6. Lu, L.; Zhang, Y.F. Influence of process control agent on interdiffusion between Al and Mg during mechanical alloying. *J. Alloy. Compd.* **1999**, *290*, 279–283. [CrossRef]
7. Miracle, D.B. Metal matrix composites—From science to technological significance. *Compos. Sci. Technol.* **2005**, *65*, 2526–2540. [CrossRef]
8. Torralba, J.M.; Da Costa, C.E.; Velasco, F. P/M aluminum matrix composites: An overview. *Proc. J. Mater. Process. Technol.* **2003**, *133*, 203–206. [CrossRef]

9. Sasaki, T.T.; Mukai, T.; Hono, K. A high-strength bulk nanocrystalline Al-Fe alloy processed by mechanical alloying and spark plasma sintering. *Scr. Mater.* **2007**, *57*, 189–192. [CrossRef]
10. Osório, W.R.; Freire, C.M.; Garcia, A. The effect of the dendritic microstructure on the corrosion resistance of Zn-Al alloys. *J. Alloy. Compd.* **2005**, *397*, 179–191. [CrossRef]
11. Ralston, K.D.; Fabijanic, D.; Birbilis, N. Effect of grain size on corrosion of high purity aluminium. *Electrochim. Acta* **2011**, *56*, 1729–1736. [CrossRef]
12. Osório, W.R.; Spinelli, J.E.; Ferreira, I.L.; Garcia, A. The roles of macrosegregation and of dendritic array spacings on the electrochemical behavior of an Al-4.5 wt.% Cu alloy. *Electrochim. Acta* **2007**, *52*, 3265–3273. [CrossRef]
13. Song, D.; Ma, A.; Jiang, J.; Lin, P.; Yang, D.; Fan, J. Corrosion behavior of equal-channel-angular-pressed pure magnesium in NaCl aqueous solution. *Corros. Sci.* **2010**, *52*, 481–490. [CrossRef]
14. Birbilis, N.; Ralston, K.D.; Virtanen, S.; Fraser, H.L.; Davies, C.H. Grain character influences on corrosion of ECAPed pure magnesium. *Corros. Eng. Sci. Technol.* **2010**, *45*, 224–230. [CrossRef]
15. Osório, W.R.; Spinelli, J.E.; Afonso, C.R.M.; Peixoto, L.C.; Garcia, A. Microstructure, corrosion behaviour and microhardness of a directionally solidified Sn-Cu solder alloy. *Electrochim. Acta* **2011**, *56*, 8891–8899. [CrossRef]
16. Son, I.J.; Nakano, H.; Oue, S.; Kobayashi, S.; Fukushima, H.; Horita, Z. Pitting corrosion resistance of ultrafine-grained aluminum processed by severe plastic deformation. *Nippon Kinzoku Gakkaishi/J. Jpn. Inst. Met.* **2006**, *47*, 1163–1169. [CrossRef]
17. Kubaski, E.T.; Cintho, O.M.; Capocchi, J.D.T. Effect of milling variables on the synthesis of NiAl intermetallic compound by mechanical alloying. *Powder Technol.* **2011**, *214*, 77–82. [CrossRef]
18. Mishra, R.; Balasubramaniam, R. Effect of nanocrystalline grain size on the electrochemical and corrosion behavior of nickel. *Corros. Sci.* **2004**, *46*, 3019–3029. [CrossRef]
19. Luo, W.; Xu, Y.; Wang, Q.; Shi, P.; Yan, M. Effect of grain size on corrosion of nanocrystalline copper in NaOH solution. *Corros. Sci.* **2010**, *52*, 3509–3513. [CrossRef]
20. Kim, S.H.; Aust, K.T.; Erb, U.; Gonzalez, F.; Palumbo, G. A comparison of the corrosion behaviour of polycrystalline and nanocrystalline cobalt. *Scr. Mater.* **2003**, *48*, 1379–1384. [CrossRef]
21. Shingu, P.H.; Huang, B.; Nishitani, S.R.; Nasu, S. Nano-meter order crystalline structure of Al-Fe alloys produced by mechanical alloying. *Suppl. Trans. JIM* **1988**, *29*, 3–10.
22. Dong, Y.D.; Wang, W.H.; Liu, L.; Xiao, K.Q.; Tong, S.H.; He, Y.Z. Structural investigation of a mechanically alloyed Al-Fe system. *Mater. Sci. Eng. A* **1991**, *134*, 867–871. [CrossRef]
23. Niu, X.P.; Froyen, L.; Delaey, L.; Peytour, C. Effect of Fe content on the mechanical alloying and mechanical properties of Al-Fe alloys. *J. Mater. Sci.* **1994**, *29*, 3724–3732. [CrossRef]
24. Nayak, S.S.; Murty, B.S.; Pabi, S.K. Structure of nanocomposites of Al-Fe alloys prepared by mechanical alloying and rapid solidification processing. *Bull. Mater. Sci.* **2008**, *31*, 449–454. [CrossRef]
25. Braun, R. Stress corrosion cracking behaviour of Al-Li alloy 8090-T8171 plate exposed to various synthetic environments. *Mater. Corros.* **2004**, *55*, 241–248. [CrossRef]
26. González-Rodríguez, J.G.; Salazar, M.; Luna-Ramírez; Porcayo-Calderon, J.; Rosas, G.; Villfane, A.M. Effect of Li, Ce and Ni on the corrosion resistance of Fe_3Al in molten Na_2SO_4 and $NaVO_3$. *High Temp. Mater. Process.* **2004**, *23*, 177–183.
27. Cai, C.; Zhang, Z.; Cao, F.; Gao, Z.; Zhang, J.; Cao, C. Analysis of pitting corrosion behavior of pure Al in sodium chloride solution with the wavelet technique. *J. Electroanal. Chem.* **2005**, *578*, 143–150. [CrossRef]
28. Gudić, S.; Smoljko, I.; Klikić, M. The effect of small addition of tin and indium on the corrosion behavior of aluminium in chloride solution. *J. Alloy. Compd.* **2010**, *505*, 54–63. [CrossRef]
29. LI, S.; Zhang, H.; LIU, J. Corrosion behavior of aluminum alloy 2024-T3 by 8-hydroxy-quinoline and its derivative in 3.5% chloride solution. *Trans. Nonferr. Met. Soc. China (Engl. Ed.)* **2007**, *17*, 318–325. [CrossRef]
30. Shen, D.; Li, G.; Guo, C.; Zou, J.; Cai, J.; He, D.; Ma, H.; Liu, F. Microstructure and corrosion behavior of micro-arc oxidation coatingon 6061 aluminum alloy pre-treated by high-temperature oxidation. *Appl. Surf. Sci.* **2013**, *287*, 451–456. [CrossRef]
31. Ralston, K.D.; Birbilis, N. Effect of grain size on corrosion: A review. *Corrosion* **2010**, *66*, 075005-075005-13. [CrossRef]

32. Gupta, R.K.; Fabijanic, D.; Zhang, R.; Birbilis, N. Corrosion behaviour and hardness of in situ consolidated nanostructured Al and Al-Cr alloys produced via high-energy ball milling. *Corros. Sci.* **2015**, *98*, 643–650. [CrossRef]
33. Sherif, E.S.M.; Ammar, H.R.; Khalil, K.A. Effects of copper and titanium on the corrosion behavior of newly fabricated nanocrystalline aluminum in natural seawater. *Appl. Surf. Sci.* **2014**, *301*, 142–148. [CrossRef]
34. Ghosh, S.K.; Dey, G.K.; Dusane, R.O.; Grover, A.K. Improved pitting corrosion behaviour of electrodeposited nanocrystalline Ni-Cu alloys in 3.0 wt.% NaCl solution. *J. Alloy. Compd.* **2006**, *426*, 235–243. [CrossRef]
35. Liu, L.; Li, Y.; Wang, F. Electrochemical corrosion behavior of nanocrystalline materials-a review. *J. Mater. Sci. Technol.* **2010**, *26*, 1–14. [CrossRef]
36. Raju, K.S.; Krishna, M.G.; Padmanabhan, K.A.; Muraleedharan, K.; Gurao, N.P.; Wilde, G. Grain size and grain boundary character distribution in ultra-fine grained (ECAP) nickel. *Mater. Sci. Eng. A* **2008**, *491*, 1–7. [CrossRef]
37. Osório, W.R.; Freire, C.M.; Garcia, A. The role of macrostructural morphology and grain size on the corrosion resistance of Zn and Al castings. *Mater. Sci. Eng. A* **2005**, *402*, 22–32. [CrossRef]
38. Cai, S.; Lei, T.; Li, N.; Feng, F. Effects of Zn on microstructure, mechanical properties and corrosion behavior of Mg-Zn alloys. *Mater. Sci. Eng. C* **2012**, *32*, 2570–2577. [CrossRef]
39. Barbucci, A.; Farnè, G.; Matteazzi, P.; Riccieri, R.; Cerisola, G. Corrosion behaviour of nanocrystalline Cu90Ni10 alloy in neutral solution containing chlorides. *Corros. Sci.* **1998**, *41*, 463–475. [CrossRef]
40. Chianpairot, A.; Lothongkum, G.; Schuh, C.A.; Boonyongmaneerat, Y. Corrosion of nanocrystalline Ni-W alloys in alkaline and acidic 3.5 wt.% NaCl solutions. *Corros. Sci.* **2011**, *53*, 1066–1071. [CrossRef]
41. Lo, P.H.; Tsai, W.T.; Lee, J.T.; Hung, M.P. Role of phosphorus in the electrochemical behavior of electroless Ni-P alloys in 3.5 wt.% NaCl solutions. *Surf. Coat. Technol.* **1994**, *67*, 27–34. [CrossRef]
42. Mote, V.D.; Purushotham, Y.; Dole, B.N. Williamson-Hall analysis in estimation of lattice strain in nanometer-sized ZnO particles. *J. Theor. Appl. Phys.* **2012**, *6*, 1–8. [CrossRef]
43. Prabhu, Y.T.; Rao, K.V.; Kumar, V.S.S.; Kumari, B.S. X-ray analysis by Williamson-Hall and size-strain plot methods of ZnO nanoparticles with fuel variation. *World J. Nano Sci. Eng.* **2014**, *4*, 21–28. [CrossRef]
44. Seikh, A.H.; Baig, M.; Ammar, H.R. Corrosion behavior of nanostructure Al-Fe alloy processed by mechanical alloying and high frequency induction heat sintering. *Int. J. Electrochem. Sci.* **2015**, *10*, 3054–3064.
45. Lee, I.S.; Kao, P.W.; Ho, N.J. Microstructure and mechanical properties of Al-Fe in situ nanocomposite produced by friction stir processing. *Intermetallics* **2008**, *16*, 1104–1108. [CrossRef]
46. Zhang, L.C.; Shen, Z.Q.; Xu, J. Glass formation in a (Ti, Zr, Hf)–(Cu, Ni, Ag)–Al high-order alloy system by mechanical alloying. *J. Mater. Res.* **2003**, *18*, 2141–2149. [CrossRef]
47. Lu, P.-J.; Huang, S.-C.; Chen, Y.-P.; Chiueh, L.-C.; Shih, D.Y.-C. Analysis of titanium dioxide and zinc oxide nanoparticles in cosmetics. *J. Food Drug Anal.* **2015**, *23*, 587–594. [CrossRef]
48. Yang, H.; Wen, J.; Quan, M.; Wang, J. Evaluation of the volume fraction of nanocrystalsdevitrified in Al-based amorphous alloys. *J. Non-Cryst. Solids* **2009**, *355*, 235–238. [CrossRef]
49. Ehtemam-Haghighi, S.; Liu, Y.; Cao, G.; Zhang, L.-C. Influence of Nb on the $\beta \rightarrow \alpha''$ martensitic phase transformation and properties of the newly designed Ti-Fe-Nb alloys. *Mater. Sci. Eng. C* **2016**, *60*, 503–510. [CrossRef]
50. Nayak, S.S.; Wollgarten, M.; Banhart, J.; Pabi, S.K.; Murty, B.S. Nanocomposites and an extremely hard nanocrystalline intermetallic of Al-Fe alloys prepared by mechanical alloying. *Mater. Sci. Eng. A* **2010**, *527*, 2370–2378. [CrossRef]
51. Basariya, M.I.R.; Mukhopadhyay, N.K. Chapter 5, Structural and mechanical behaviour of Al-Fe intermetallics. In *Intermetallics Compounds*; IntechOpen: London, UK, 2018. [CrossRef]
52. Keong, P.G.; Sames, J.A.; Adam, C.M.; Sharp, R.M. Influence of various elements on Al-Al_6Fe eutectic system. In Proceedings of the International Conference on Solidification and Casting of Metals, London, UK, 18–21 July 1977; pp. 110–114.
53. Campbell, J. *Castings*; Butterworth-Heinemann: Oxford, MS, UK, 2003.
54. Seri, O.; Tagashira, K. The interpretation of polarization curves for A1-Fe alloys in de-aerated NaCl solution. *Corros. Sci.* **1990**, *30*, 87–94. [CrossRef]
55. Liang, J.; Gao, L.J.; Miao, N.N.; Chai, Y.J.; Wang, N.; Song, X.Q. Hydrogen generation by reaction of Al-M(M = Fe, Co, Ni) with water. *Energy* **2016**, *113*, 282–287. [CrossRef]

56. Grosjean, M.H.; Zidoune, M.; Roue, L. Hydrogen production from highly corroding Mg-based materials elaborated by ball milling. *J. Alloy. Compd.* **2005**, *404*, 712–715. [CrossRef]
57. Flores-Chan, J.E.; Bedolla-Jacuinde, A.; Patiño-Carachure, C.; Rosas, G.; Espinosa-Medina, M.A. Corrosion study of Al-Fe (20 wt-%) alloy in artificial sea water with NaOH additions. *Can. Metall. Q.* **2018**, *57*, 201–209. [CrossRef]
58. Seri, O.; Furumata, K. Effect of Al-Fe-Si intermetallic compound phases on initiation and propagation of pitting attacks for aluminum 1100. *Mater. Corros.* **2002**, *53*, 111–120. [CrossRef]
59. Dean, S.W. Electrochemical methods of corrosion testing. In *Electrochemical Techniques for Corrosion*; Baboian, R., Ed.; NACE: Houston, TX, USA, 1977; p. 52.
60. Pariona, M.; Micene, K.T.; Zara, J. Effect of microstructure on microhardness and electrochemical behavior in hypereutectic Al-Fe alloy processed by laser surface remelting. In *Aerospace Engineering*; IntechOpen: London, UK, 2019. [CrossRef]
61. Sherif, E.M.; Park, S.M. Effects of 1,4-naphthoquinone on aluminum corrosion in 0.50 M sodium chloride solutions. *Electrochim. Acta* **2006**, *51*, 1313–1321. [CrossRef]
62. Ma, H.; Chen, S.; Niu, L.; Zhao, S.; Li, S.; Li, D. Inhibition of copper corrosion by several Schiff bases in aerated halide solutions. *J. Appl. Electrochem.* **2002**, *32*, 65–72. [CrossRef]
63. Singh, A.K.; Shukla, S.K.; Singh, M.; Quraishi, M.A. Inhibitive effect of ceftazidime on corrosion of mild steel in hydrochloric acid solution. *Mater. Chem. Phys.* **2011**, *129*, 68–76. [CrossRef]
64. Sherif, E.M.; Park, S.M. Effects of 2-amino-5-ethylthio-1,3,4-thiadiazole on copper corrosion as a corrosion inhibitor in aerated acidic pickling solutions. *Electrochim. Acta* **2006**, *51*, 6556–6562. [CrossRef]
65. Rehim, S.S.A.; Hassan, H.H.; Amin, M.A. Corrosion and corrosion inhibition of Al and some alloys in sulphate solutions containing halide ions investigated by an impedance technique. *Appl. Surf. Sci.* **2002**, *187*, 279–290. [CrossRef]
66. Zhou, Y.L.; Niinomi, M.; Akahori, T.; Fukui, H.; Toda, H. Corrosion resistance and biocompatibility of Ti-Ta alloys for biomedical applications. *Mater. Sci. Eng. A* **2005**, *398*, 28–36. [CrossRef]
67. Seri, O. The effect of NaCl concentration on the corrosion behavior of Aluminum containing iron. *Corros. Sci.* **1994**, *36*, 1789–1803. [CrossRef]
68. Gupta, R.K.; Birbilis, N. The influence of nanocrystalline structure and processing route on corrosion of stainless steel: A review. *Corros. Sci.* **2015**, *92*, 1–15. [CrossRef]
69. Frankel, G.S. On the pitting resistance of sputter-deposited aluminum alloys. *J. Electrochem. Soc.* **1993**, *140*, 2192–2197. [CrossRef]

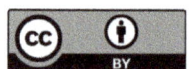

© 2019 by the authors. Licensee MDPI, Basel, Switzerland. This article is an open access article distributed under the terms and conditions of the Creative Commons Attribution (CC BY) license (http://creativecommons.org/licenses/by/4.0/).

MDPI
St. Alban-Anlage 66
4052 Basel
Switzerland
Tel. +41 61 683 77 34
Fax +41 61 302 89 18
www.mdpi.com

Coatings Editorial Office
E-mail: coatings@mdpi.com
www.mdpi.com/journal/coatings

www.ingramcontent.com/pod-product-compliance
Lightning Source LLC
LaVergne TN
LVHW070607100526
838202LV00012B/584